Truth or Consequences

A New Vision for
Health and Healing

To Mel –
May your life be
full of Joy.
Love,
Jack Becker J mo

TRUTH OR CONSEQUENCES

A NEW VISION FOR HEALTH AND HEALING

BY
JASPER B. BECKER, JR., M.D.

Jasper B. Becker, Jr., M.D.
2909 Banchory Road
Winter Park, FL 32792
Telephone: (407) 657-8044
Fax: (407) 657-8419
Email: jbbmd@parkave.net

Printed in the United States of America.

ISBN 0-9664194-0-5

To
Loren

Thanks.
See you later, dude.

"*Truth or Consequences* is a powerful, insightful, easy to read book, written from the heart, that will help set a new vision for healing–for both the physician and the patient. BRAVO!"

Gerald G. Jampolsky, M.D., Founder, Center for Attitudinal Healing and best-selling author of *Love is Letting Go of Fear* and other books.

"It was a pleasure to read *Truth or Consequences* by Jasper Becker, M.D. His warmth as a human, his dedication as a physician, and his openness as a spiritual being create the powerful ambience of this volume. How refreshing it is to see the healing process through wholeness-oriented eyes of this exceptional physician. We are invited on an extraordinarily engrossing journey for the mind, body, and spirit which is punctuated by absorbing personal experiences and case examples."

Deirdre Davis Brigham, M.S., MPH, MA
Fellow & Diplomate, American Board of Medical Psychotherapists; Author, *Imagery for Getting Well: Clinical Applications of Behavioral Medicine* (W.W. Norton, 1994)

TABLE OF CONTENTS

ACKNOWLEDGEMENTS

Thanks to my parents for having me and giving me the freedom to find my own way, even though this must have been painful at times. Thanks to Kathy for helping me gradually move out of my head and into my heart, and for showing me that having a friend is more important than sticking to my schedule.

Thanks to my children for helping me understand the importance of unconditional love.

Thanks to Attitudinal Healing which is taking away my need to fix, and is showing me the importance of simply listening.

Thanks to Deirdre Brigham, Getting Well, Inc., and the return group for being my support system and learning arena, as we have attempted together to look deeper into the meaning of healing.

Thanks to Diane London for special editing, and all those friends and family who have read my manuscript and offered advice, corrections, inspiration and encouragement to proceed.

Thanks to Jane Harrington, whose artwork symbolizes to me the coming out of our self-imposed limits into the dawning of enlightenment, exemplified by the rising sun on the lovely cover, and the going within oneself as in the *Crab Trap* illustrations.

Thanks to Josh McCloud for the imaginative illustrations of the *Dave the Wave* story.

Thanks to Cat Sanders for her light-hearted personality and her business-like expertise in putting it all together and getting this material into print.

AUTHOR'S NOTE

Writing this book has been an exercise in clarifying my own thoughts about healing. At times, I wonder why I am publishing this material, and to whom I think it might appeal. Then someone reads what I have written and gains insight into his or her own healing potential, and I am encouraged to proceed.

I do not claim to be a scientist, for I see these gifted people as dedicated researchers, striving toward absolute answers. Even though I have had years of experience in the practice of the science and healing art of medicine, I have often been perplexed at the success or failure of my own healing efforts. I have never found any consistency in the explanations, and am content in simply not needing to know all the answers.

I am not a trained psychotherapist or psychologist, but have long-term experience in observing psycho-biological responses in patients.

It is in the arena of beliefs and attitudes, that uncertain, unscientific, constantly changing stage located in the mind somewhere between the light of Truth and the darkness of fear, that I feel most comfortable and alive. I have come to enjoy listening, waiting, watching, sometimes probing and prodding, and observing with wonder as a shift in consciousness occurs. With patience and trust, somehow the light creeps in, the impossible is made possible, and the unexpected is experienced, accepted, and embraced as the new norm.

There are large numbers of people who have naively accepted the belief that healing comes from somewhere outside themselves. It is for them that this book is written. I hope it will open a doorway for them to become aware of, and be empowered by, their own Inner Healer.

FOREWORD

by Gerald G. Jampolsky, M.D.

This is a powerful book that speaks from the heart that has the potential for helping transform how we physicians practice medicine, and how patients can participate and take responsibility for the process. Dr. Becker shares with great honesty his own spiritual transformation process, and emphasizes the need to heal our own spirit and our mind—as a part of the healing process. He sees our true identity as a spiritual one. He goes on to suggest that as we heal our minds and the hole in our soul, we can experience ourselves as whole. He eloquently describes the importance of the forgiveness process.

Truth or Consequences is a courageous book filled with many personal anecdotes which makes for both easy and illuminating reading. As we approach the 21st Century, this book is an exciting bridge for all of us to take a new look at what healing is all about.

INTRODUCTION

Would you like to walk through life feeling confident and unafraid? Would you like to feel healthy and know you are in control of your own sense of well-being? These goals are achievable without buying anything or joining anything. Its only cost is giving up illusions that blind you, and removing the self-imposed chains that bind you.

Focusing on the healing arts, we take a look at the present state of health care from the perspective of a physician who has been in medical practice in a variety of settings for 36 years. What is revealed is a medical care system which has an unclear objective, striving for goals that are unattainable. A major transition is gradually occurring as basic concepts are changing regarding life, death, disease, health, and healing.

This transition is interconnected with changes occurring throughout our society. Huge foundational belief system shifts are reshaping our basic concepts. Long accepted theories are being replaced by new knowledge that calls for a totally different model of the world, of life, and of time-space reality.

For several hundred years the concrete reality of the physical sciences has been our touchstone of truth, where we have placed our hope to improve the lot of humanity. Even though spectacular progress has occurred, something central in our approach is obviously missing, because we are still grappling with the same old problems of despair, disease, sadness, suffering, starvation, crime, war, etc. Also, we are creating new problems such as previously unknown diseases, toxic pollution, depletion of natural resources, and environmental destruction.

We desperately need to find a more valid truth, a cornerstone on which to build our future.

We are living in a world and a society whose motivations and decisions are primarily based on fear. These fear oriented decisions adversely affect each of us and all of our institutions, including our health care system. This book looks at the effect this system has had on the patient. It describes the patient's frustrations at being depersonalized, being seen as an illness, a statistic, or an economic unit, rather than as a distinctive, total individual with a personality, feelings and soul. The book empowers the patient who may experience helplessness in the face of disease and urges him/her take a responsible role in the healing process.

This book also presents a voice for the medical doctors and other health care providers who may, likewise, feel frustrated, discounted, disenchanted and oppressed by a medical system which has become so entangled in scientific statistical analysis, bureaucracy, politics and economics that it has been side-tracked from its original humanitarian goal of facilitating healing.

The roles of mind, consciousness, and spirituality emerge in prominence and take their rightful place in the healing process. The painful steps of my own stretch of consciousness are described, which has resulting in a radical shift of my thinking. Whereas only a few short years ago my mind was totally scientifically oriented and closed, now I am comfortable with a view which recognizes an infinitely wider range of possibilities.

Many personal experiences and medical case reports are presented illustrating the interconnectedness of emotional and spiritual health with physical well-being. These demonstrate how our beliefs and our thoughts influence both the development of disease, and the recovery from it. There is an understandable explanation of the immune system and how it responds to our beliefs, thoughts and feelings.

The definition of disease is expanded to include not only physical infirmities, but mental, emotional, and spiritual imbalances as well. These imbalances are seen not only in the individual, but are shown to exist also in our relationships, our society, and our environment. It is suggested that if we first create balance within our hearts and minds, then we will create healthy bodies, relationships, and societies.

The philosophical heart of this book addresses humankind's fundamental question, "Who are we?" Is identifying ourselves only as physical bodies an error in our belief system which dooms us? We look at how body identification has effected us individually and collectively as a society, and how it influences the health care profession. This book leads us on a search for a better way to define ourselves, and shows us how this can dramatically change our lives and our potential for healing.

This book illustrates how, through guilt, fear, intimidation and rationalization, we block the intimacy of truly knowing ourselves and each other. It instructs us on removing the masks which hide our feelings; on untangling the web of our internal deceptions; on experiencing unconditional forgiveness; and thus reclaiming our true identity. The result is an awakening to a concept of our greater reality, allowing us to experience the true healing that we have been missing, which penetrates deeply, all the way through our souls.

SECTION
1

Identifying
The
Problem

CHAPTER 1

PERSONAL
BACKGROUND

I have introduced an idea that the system of medical care is in a state of transition, hopefully to something better. My opinions relating to the scientifically oriented medical system evolved during the 38 years that I have been in medical training and practice. Those involving quantum physics, metaphysics and spirituality, subjects which are vital to the changing medical paradigm as I see it, are of more recent origin.

I was born the only boy and middle child of a stable, middle class family in south Mississippi in 1934. I was surrounded by loving relatives and experienced the real meaning of extended family. An early motivation toward a medical career was implanted by my grandfather and uncle who were physicians, as well as by the devoted care given me during some serious illnesses by a kindly family physician. His primary tools, at a time prior to the availability of antibiotics, were the magic of his presence and his knowledge and practice of the healing art of medicine. My parents encouraged me toward a professional career because they had lived through the depression and understood the value of having a means of livelihood which would offer financial security even during the worst of times.

World War II filled my youth, and even though our family was affected by losses, I remember these times more like a glorious "good guys against the bad guys" adventure of heroism, and of course the good guys eventually won. When the war ended, I was eleven years old and my world view was totally black and white with no confusing shades of gray. It was great to be an American. It was obvious to me that if only everyone else could accept our values and views, then the whole human race could be as happy as we were!

The experiences of Catholic grade school, then public junior high and high school imprinted themselves deeply on my developing psyche. Some of these impressions were helpful and some were limiting. Many friends, social activities, athletics, and a loving home environment all contributed to making these quite memorable years, and many times I have felt a longing for the past, when life choices seemed much simpler.

Emotionally, I was quite immature when I left home for college, but I somehow managed to graduate from Washington and Lee University. Like many college students, my focus was not entirely on formal education. I was determined to taste a little of all that life had to offer. By the time I entered Tulane Medical School I was married and we were expecting our first child. She was born in the early morning, just a few hours before my first Gross Anatomy exam. The fact that I managed to pass this test under these trying circumstances gave me renewed confidence in my ability to get through medical school successfully. My delight at having an adorable daughter increased my resolve to work toward a dignified and financially secure profession.

Medical school was a very fearful, intense, traumatic emotional experience. I was insecure and fearful of failure. At first, I felt unworthy to be there, and harbored paranoid fears that the authorities would soon discover they had made a mistake in admitting me. My memories are like a giant collage including images of trying to learn how to make married life a happy experience, having babies, the stench of cadavers soaking in formaldehyde, all night study sessions, Mardi Gras, Phi Chi fraternity parties, Bull Pen, the loss of a child, bridge games, grades, decisions about career, all in a chaotic pattern with little meaning, leading nowhere in particular other than to some distant glorious day when the training would be completed and I could really start living.

I was very impressionable and introverted, and as we studied each disease I was certain that I had it. At one time or another I remember being convinced I was suffering from heart disease, stomach ulcers, cancer, diabetes, tuberculosis, lupus, syphilis, leukemia and other terrifying illnesses.

I was graduated from medical school without any particular honor or dishonor, but just the relief of completing the process was reward in itself. I am proud of one particular achievement: being elected medical school student body president my senior year. I must have been pretty good at hiding all my insecurities to be voted this honor. Probably, everyone else had been experiencing these same feelings and felt I was a valid representative for them.

I made it through a nightmarish year as an intern at Charity Hospital in New Orleans. It was a "rotating" internship, which meant spending time in different specialty areas. My first rotation was in Internal Medicine. I had chosen this because I was intellectually attracted to diagnostic problem solving. I thought perhaps this specialty would offer that opportunity. There was an urgency to make an early decision regarding specialization and to apply for a residency position for the next year, so I wanted to investigate Internal Medicine first.

I was assigned two "colored" male wards and one "white" male ward. This numbered about 60 beds in all, and they were all full. There was minimal staff supervision, and the responsibility for the total care of these patients was delegated to one first year Internal Medicine resident and myself. My memory is one of complete chaos and exhaustion. I remember that too many people died, and I felt helpless to save them. Many were beyond hope when they were admitted. Some improved, but others got worse under our care. There was no time for the studious, pipe-smoking, intellectualizing which I had envisioned Internal Medicine to be.

I began to look for a surgical specialty because I was hopeful that surgery could more definitively correct problems and offer more hope for a cure. Urology appealed to me because it offered excellent diagnostic tools which usually made it possible to make a specific diagnosis before surgery.

I was accepted as a resident in Urology at Ochsner Foundation Hospital. Residency was a difficult and humbling learning experience with intensive demands from the staff, very long hours, and very little time at home. It seemed as though there was never enough time to do a thorough job at anything. I was constantly running from one urgent problem to another with no time for serious study or contemplation.

I honestly do not know what drove me to complete all these years of training. Probably it was fear of failure. I know now in hindsight that I was not enjoying the experience, and I have blocked out much of my memory of the emotional trauma. There are still flashbacks that wake me up in a cold sweat. However, it was exciting and kept my adrenaline flowing. I think the feeling was much like that of soldiers going through extremely traumatic battle experiences. I was feeling the excitement of fully participating in life, with its exhilarating, boundary-expanding highs, interspersed with periods of total frustration and exhaustion. The thought of quitting never entered my mind as there seemed to be no other options.

Life was going on around us, but I hardly remember it. When time permitted, social events were usually occasions to unwind from all the tension, drink to excess and to "let it all hang out."

The hectic, absurd, and compulsive life style of my medical training must have allowed at least a little time at home. My wife and I had brought five children into the world by the time the residency was completed. My wife, undoubtedly exhausted and exasperated, faithfully stuck by me, even though I had little time to give toward marriage and family life. Many problems in our relationship were swept under the rug, awaiting some imaginary future period when we would have the time and maturity to deal with them.

My medical training had been consistent with what I believe was generally the standard for the day. By that I mean that it focused primarily on the physical treatment of physical illness. The general medical philosophy I learned was to be detached from the patient, find the physical cause of the disease as directly as possible, and prescribe the proper treatment. The doctor that could "find it and fix it" most rapidly was held in highest esteem. It reminds me of the parlor game, Twenty Questions: Find the answer with as few questions as possible. Of course, this did not allow time to inquire much about how the patient was feeling emotionally, or about other factors in his life, such as his relationships, his job, his fears, his ambitions and his disappointments.

I think most of my fellow students were convinced, as I was, that this detached, unemotional approach was correct. There seemed to be an unwritten understanding that "they" were the patients and "we" were the healers. We were supposed to know what was best for them, and their opinion did not count for much. We needed to maintain an air of authority. It was considered unwise to become emotionally involved by getting too close to their feelings. Hopefully medical schools are changing. Frankly, I haven't observed much difference in the philosophy of more recent graduates, who continue to pursue the diagnosis and treatment of illness in the same limited, arms-length fashion.

There was limited exposure to psychiatric theory and training, but at least we learned to identify some mental and emotional illnesses. The scientific focus regarding mental illness was, as I recall, that there were chemical, genetic and structural abnormalities in the brain that underlay mental diseases. The consensus was that with time, research would solve all of these problems.

The thing of most value that I remember from that brief psychiatric exposure was my introduction to the idea of psychosomatic illnesses. I was impressed that psychological problems could show up as physical symptoms. It was suggested, for example, that persons in stressful jobs might be prone to stomach ulcers, or that excessive worry might cause headaches. Unfortunately, there was no teaching of stress management at that time, and in spite of a general understanding of that "mind-body" connection, therapy was aimed primarily at the ulcer or the headache instead of at the underlying stress. This treatment at the effect level remains the standard way of handling these and similar problems today. The causal level of the creation and treatment of illness is just now coming into focus.

When my formal medical training had finally come to an end with the completion of my residency in 1965, I moved to Pensacola, Florida, and joined the private practice of two established Urologists. I was 33, finally on the verge of earning a decent wage for the first time in my life, when Uncle Sam expressed a desire for me to serve as an "obligatory volunteer" in the U. S. Army Medical Corp. Although shocked at this upheaval, I was secretly excited about the opportunity because I had become disenchanted by some unexpected developments in my medical practice and was also quite perplexed about my marriage. To escape from an unhappy situation and to experience a new adventure was appealing. Going into the Army for two years was, in some ways, a relief.

I learned a lot in the Army, but most of what I took away was not what the army was trying to teach me. My experiences during a year with the 93rd Evacuation Hospital in Vietnam were gruesome at times, but some were rewarding, exciting, and occasionally even fun. I remember that I could tell how bad the mass casualty situation was by the intensity of the red color of the water in the drainage ditch outside the operating room building. I can still vividly remember the disparaging sight of mangled bodies and severed limbs lying on the floor of the operating room, and the distressing feeling of being elbow deep in blood as we tried to stem the flow before another young life had slipped away.

Strangely, one of my most vivid memories is the voice of Martin Luther King on the radio in the triage area as we were frantically busy in a mass casualty situation. Reverend King was expressing his opinion against America's involvement in this ghastly war, stating forcefully, "Stop the bombing! Stop the bombing!" How strange it seemed to be able to consider that stopping our side of the war might be a solution, while at the same time taking care of the bloody results of vicious attacks by the enemy. By the time that year was over, I wasn't at all sure just who the enemy was. I thought the war in Vietnam was a horrible waste of lives on both sides.

There was pathos as well as humor, and I appreciate the TV series "MASH" and "China Beach" for giving moving an accurate portrayals of many of these military hospitals.

After my obligatory two years in the military, I felt a renewed determination to try to be a good husband and father, and to raise my family in an environment that would be safe, free and loving. I went back to the town of my birth, Brookhaven, Mississippi, and opened a solo practice in Urology in 1968.

I could write a separate book about the next 16 years which were full of successes, failures, trials, tribulations, grief and happiness. There remain many lasting friendships and wonderful memories that I will always cherish.

For much of that time I was the only Urologist in an area extending from New Orleans, Louisiana and Jackson, Mississippi on the south and north, and Natchez and Hattiesburg, Mississippi west and east, and developed a successful practice through the support and cooperation of many fine physicians.

We had one more child during that period who has been a real blessing. Her mother and I, sadly, however, eventually came to the unspoken knowing that our marriage was over.

Sometimes it helps to laugh when one is telling about something that is painful, so I will tell the following story of my departure, which was later humorously referred to as "The Great Escape" by a neighbor who was my friend, confidant, lawyer, and sporting companion.

My wife and I had agreed that I would move out of the house quietly on a Monday morning while the children were at school. I had been living in a downstairs bedroom for quite some time and had the few possessions I needed all packed and ready to go.

I rented a U-Haul truck and wheeled into my driveway at about 9:00 AM. I had failed to notice there was a large cable hanging over the driveway which supported the electrical wires and the telephone line. This cable was fairly high and had never been a problem for an automobile, but the truck had a much higher body. The truck snagged the cable, pulling down a telephone pole on one end, and a part of the side of the house on the other! My secret departure was immediately exposed. Very shortly the yard was filled with workmen from the electric company and the telephone company, plus neighbors from all sides. They all ended up helping me load the truck, and waved good-bye as I drove away. It must have been very amusing to those observing, but I felt defeated, deflated and embarrassed. I was determined, however, to escape from a situation which I felt powerless to change, and for which I had not the mental and emotional tools to sustain further.

I do not wish to make my divorce appear to be something that I took lightly. I was emotionally devastated by the whole lengthy process, which had taken years to come to a con-clusion. In my mind I had made a commitment that this was a lifelong union, and being the permanent father in a large and loving family was also a vision that I assumed would last a lifetime. When that proved beyond the limited capabilities of my first wife and me to attain, I felt a deep sense of loss and disappointment.

I managed to survive the loneliness of the separation and the challenges of bachelorhood. My ex-wife did an admirable job of being single again for the first time since she was 17 years old. We are both remarried, relocated, communicating better than in the past, and living productive lives. My second wife, Kathy, whom I married a year after my divorce, is a joy and a cherished companion. In our marriage, now in its 15th year, we have each been teacher and student for the other. Our children have adjusted, working through and acting out some major anger and disappointment. Going through this was not easy, and we were forced to make some difficult decisions.

In 1985 Kathy and I decided to give in to our long-standing urge to move to Florida. We selected Orlando because it appeared cosmopolitan, exciting and seemed to provide professional opportunities.

I had been practicing in Orlando for three years when my most tragically significant, life-changing experience occurred. Kathy's daughter, Loren Quinn, whom I emotionally considered to be my daughter as well, was killed in an auto accident. She was fourteen. This was a severe and depressing blow and it certainly affected my emotions and my thought processes in many ways. I will discuss this in more detail later, but the end result was that I gradually lost interest in continuing in active surgical practice. I retired from private practice after three more years, this time for the purpose of pursuing a new-found interest in a broader definition of healing.

After almost a year of study and contemplation, an opportunity presented itself to work part-time for the Veterans Administration, practicing Urology in an outpatient clinic. I signed on, and for two years had some very interesting and rewarding experiences trying to understand and meet the needs of the veterans. This turned out to be an opportunity to gain some insight into another facet of the medical system of this country.

I am now retired from active private medical practice but am still involved in the healing profession through *Getting Well, Inc.*,[1] a not-for-profit, behavioral medical facility in Orlando. The focus here is offering patients with life challenging or chronic debilitating illnesses a safe place where, under professional guidance, they can look deeply into their own beliefs, thoughts and behavior patterns. In so doing, they are empowered to take control of the healing resources within themselves. Of all the experiences I have had in the medical profession, this is proving to be the most exciting. I feel that I am finally learning what healing is all about.

This chapter has been about my own personal history, and I will end with the following story, because I believe the experience I will describe helped me view my life from a more positive perspective. This is important to me, as I have a tendency toward a neurotic personality which generally focuses on the negative. It was my first experience with journaling, which I have since come to appreciate as a powerful psychological tool.

My step son, Rafe Quinn, then about 12 years old, was given an assignment in his English class to compile a book of his family history. He asked his grandparents, uncles and aunts, his mother, and also me, to write a summary of our lives.

I remember that I was honored when he asked me to do this, but at the time I was not feeling positive about my past. Two of my daughters were experiencing difficulties in their lives, and in accordance with my usual pattern, I was feeling guilty because I thought I had not been as responsive as I could have been as a parent. I could think of all sorts of things that I could have or should have said or done which probably would have given them different life skills. Along with the guilt, I was angry because they did not care for my advice and I also assumed they were blaming me for their problems. This fit right into my pattern of feeling overly responsible, even guilty because I had not lived up to my image of a parent who was always supposed to know what was best for his children.

This self-flagellating feeling of guilt, and the resulting angry feelings bothered me for several days in spite of all the intellectual arguments that I could muster against it. Finally, very early one morning of a restless night, I decided that writing about my feelings might help. I chose to use the new word processor even though I wasn't very familiar with its many functions.

I went back to my earliest memories and wrote down exactly how I felt at the present moment about every incident from my past in which I remembered feeling guilty, angry, threatened, hurt, jealous, insulted, frightened, intimidated, or irresponsible, especially those times when I had done or said nothing about these feelings.

My natural tendency had always been to suppress and even deny my feelings. There was a lot that I had "stuffed" into my subconscious mind. Apparently it was time for me to bring it up again and look at it. Well! This uninhibited writing turned out to be quite an experience, and the words came pouring out.

Some of the language surprised me as I expressed things I had been too "nice" to say publicly. The time passed quickly and before I knew it, six hours had gone by. I had left no stone unturned. Every unpleasant feeling of my life that I could remember had at last come out and been expressed. My typing gradually came to a halt as I ran out of feelings that needed to be exposed.

I touched the Escape key on my computer to conclude the typing. Much to my amazement, a question appeared on the monitor which asked, "Do you want to save this information?" The only choices given for an answer were "YES" or "NO."

Wow! I rocked back in my chair in stunned silence for a few moments. I decided the only possible answer was "NO." I pressed the "N" key and six hours of emotion-driven typing disappeared from my computer memory. Metaphorically, but quite realistically, at the same instant a lifetime of stored anguish disappeared from my emotional memory banks. I could literally feel a very heavy weight lift from my shoulders!

I am still in awe over how easy it was to let go of all of that "stuff," and how such a simple decision in my mind could have such a profound, instantaneous effect on my emotions and sense of well-being. I know now, absolutely, that I can choose which segments of the past I want to keep and allow to influence my life, and which I can choose to let go.

The next day, I wrote the requested biography for my son, and it was filled with happy experiences and with gratitude for so many good things in my life, which I had not been able to see while the clouds of my grievances were blocking my view. Thank you, Rafe, for giving me this opportunity!

Chapter 2

My View From The Inside The Medical System

I have spent more than half my life in the health care system. I have observed major transitions in this system from the viewpoint of a variety of practice settings. Never, during this time, has the practice of medicine been more confusing or more burdened with frustrating baggage than it is now.

If one looks only at scientific progress and the technical improvements in the health care system, it would be difficult to see anything but tremendous progress. Compared to what was available when I trained and started practice, there have been vast changes. The information obtained from a CT scan or an MRI study gives us information that was previously unavailable without exploratory surgery. Laboratories have machines which can perform analysis of 50 or more components of the blood in a matter of minutes. Operating rooms are a marvel of technology, which is ever changing and advancing. Ultrasound procedures give us answers about everything from the sex of a fetus to blood flow through arteries and veins, and can even destroy kidney stones. There are fascinating nuclear medical studies and treatments, using radioactive substances biologically targeted for particular body sites. Intravascular diagnostic studies and procedures using tiny flexible wires and tubes, balloon dilators, lasers, blocking devices, and chemicals can locate and treat problems throughout the body. Flexible fiberoptic instruments allow endoscopic viewing and surgery of remote parts of the body without making external incisions. Surgery is often performed through small button hole incisions, and repairs are made and entire organs removed by the skillful use of innovative surgical instruments while viewing internally using micro-television cameras. We have organ transplants of all varieties, even including the heart, and now, through genetic engineering and cloning we appear on the threshold of growing new organs in the laboratory. There are hundreds of more powerful antibiotics, antihypertensives, tranquilizers, antidepressants, pain relievers, and many other pills for the treatment of just about any abnormal condition that a patient could have.

This list only scratches the surface of inventive improvements in the huge arsenal available for medical diagnosis and treatment. Impressive also are the spaciousness, decor, and cleanliness, and efficiency of new medical facilities.

We should be rejoicing, but for some reason there seems to be a groundswell of discontent and frustration in the minds of both health care recipients and providers. Where is the problem? What are we missing? Could it be that we are so dazzled by our successes that we are unable to see our short-comings?

In the past, when there were not so many options, patients seemed much more accepting of the fact that life included disease and death. Doctors seemed to know the limits of what the medical care system had to offer. Patients took care of many things themselves, not showing up in the doctors office for every bout of nervous indigestion, or in the emergency room for every bump on the head.

Now, with so much information readily available to the public on the hazards of just about everything that we do, our attention is constantly focused on danger and disease. This feeds our fear and promotes our feelings of helplessness. To the rescue come the wonderful promises of the health care industry. Government directives, bulletins from distinguished medical associations, and advertisements from the huge, free market medical-industrial complex inform us of the diverse, and often conflicting treatment options available which promise protection and relief from all these fearful realities which surround us and afflict us.

A Setup For Codependency

There has always been a relationship between the public and the health care system in which one depended on the other. It might be stated thusly: "You help me with my health needs, and, in turn, I will assist you with your financial needs." In the past, this arrangement was practical and based on reasonable understanding and shared responsibility. The patient did what he could for himself before seeking professional assistance, and realized that there was a limit on what to expect from the medical care-giver. Treatment options were limited, cure was not promised, and fees demanded were affordable.

Times changed. An unhealthy relationship developed between patients and the medical care industry. Patients became so fearful of disease, both actual and imagined, and frustrated with the many difficult choices, that they completely gave away their responsibility for health to the health care system. The medical care system agreed to take on this impossible burden and did their best, but the cost has become enormous.

This arrangement is not working, neither party is happy, and adjustments are in progress.

The Changing Patient

In the mind of the average patient, thoughts of health are clouded by fear and uncertainty. There has been a loss of trust and faith in the system. Many patients are disenchanted, even angry at the system, which they perceive as having failed them after they come to believe that scientific health care was a guarantee for perpetual good health. They are waking up to the grim but realistic fact that, in spite of marvelous technological advances, our health care system does not have all the answers. They are also frustrated and frightened at the escalating cost of this medical care arrangement which they have bought into. Also, and perhaps most deeply disappointing of all, they have experienced the increasingly impersonal nature of modern health care.

Patients are growing tired of playing the role of the helpless victim and are realizing they can no longer afford this luxury. Somewhat begrudgingly the public is facing up to the reality that they can take some responsibility for their own health maintenance and disease prevention. Through self education many are finding encouragement. They are seeing the results of better nutrition, exercise, and lifestyle changes. They are beginning to understand also that they not only can prevent some illnesses, but that they have some control over their own healing mechanism. This discovery is empowering, and many wish to have even more involvement in their own treatment.

It is encouraging to see this change emerging. Instead of blocking or discouraging patients from gaining information and investigating alternative treatments, some medical establishments as well as individual practitioners are supporting and assisting them in making informed decisions, and welcome their responsible involvement in health choices.

The Changing Role Of Health Care Provider

Let us examine some specific problematic areas within our present system of providing optimal scientific medical care. Most clearly visible is the economic issue. We can no longer afford the cost. The health care system is teetering on the edge of financial bankruptcy. In our affluent society there are great numbers of people receiving inadequate medical attention purely because of a shortage of funds, both individually and in the government treasury. Everyone jokes about the fact that the first question one is asked when entering a hospital or practitioner's office, is not "How can we help you?" but "How will you be paying for your care?"

Such cynicism gives rise to the question of possible moral bankruptcy. Perhaps it is time to look at exactly which parts of our medical care system we are valuing, and which parts we are neglecting. We are spending a huge portion of the available health care dollar on extremely expensive, high-technology machines, on cost-intensive treatments like organ transplants and massive last-ditch chemotherapy, and on long-term, financially depleting life support for numerous patients who are essentially lifeless and who have no reasonable chance for recovery. At the same time, thousands of our citizens die or become chronically disabled for lack of treatment of less complicated illnesses because they lack access to the medical system, usually traceable to economic deficiency. As a result, one could speculate that the emphasis of our present system is geared toward prolonging the lives of the wealthy and supporting the financial well-being of the Medical-Technological-Pharmacological industry rather than focusing on raising the level of health of the general population.

PHYSICIANS

Almost any group of American physicians could come to consensus on the problems facing medical practice today. I doubt if many of these groups could come to agreement on solutions to the problems.

Many doctors are frustrated and exhausted by the demands of the present system and disenchanted by the lack of personal satisfaction. Every effort to change the system through new rules and regulations seems to lead to even more confusion. Out of desperation, many physicians are reexamining their own motivations and commitment. This feeling of a lack of fulfillment is motivating a renewed philosophical search for meaning. It is from this inner searching that solutions will arise, one physician at a time, until their commonality is realized and the system itself is changed.

The life of a physician during this period of rapidly changing and expanding scientific medicine has been exciting, but also quite humbling. The age of the "generalist" passed, and the huge amount of new information has forced doctors to specialize and even sub-specialize into ever shrinking comfort zones of expertise. This diminishes one's confidence in his general healing capabilities. It is also isolating, and one tends to develop tunnel vision and lose the overall view of the depth and breadth of the healing profession.

In addition, most physicians did not receive training in financial matters. In the past, doctors were quite well rewarded financially, and most people felt deservatively so, without the need for much expertise in the fields of economic inventiveness and financial planning. In the new climate of intense competition for the medical dollar, many physicians are recognizing their deficiencies in the ever shifting financial arena, and are understandably fearful of the loss of income and financial stability. Many are taking business courses which there wasn't time for during premedical college days, or even returning to college for an MBA.

The average physician is now finding himself with fewer patients, more rules and regulations that require more employees, and escalating costs of equipment, wages, health insurance, and especially medical liability insurance. He may be in the uncomfortable position of being forced to advertise, (something that was considered unethical only a few years ago), or to sell out his independence to some managed-care organization. Just to stay even financially, he must see more patients, spending less quality, caregiving time with each, and thus adding to his own and the patients frustration.

In the increasingly impersonal environment of medical care, it sometimes seems, from the patient's viewpoint at least, that the profit incentive is all that matters to the health care providers. The cost of medical care has certainly become astonishingly high, and this care is regarded by many patients as of lower value in terms of human concern, kindness, and compassion.

Many physicians are fighting against this system which they find intolerable, and through their efforts alternative ways of practicing quality medicine are emerging.

There are, of course, still many physicians who truly enjoy their profession and feel adequately rewarded. Thank Heaven for these, as they seem to have found an island of stability amid a stormy sea, and we need their equanimity.

Some physicians simply enjoy the pleasure of mastering technical skills, and I see nothing wrong with that. Some of the most highly skilled surgeons and some of the most adept diagnosticians enjoy the purely technical and scientifically challenging aspects of medicine.

One problem that is being addressed in the changing medical system is equitable compensation for those physicians who prefer care-giving to technology. It is becoming appreciated that time spent listening to patients is healing in itself, and in modern economic terms is "cost effective." A patient's greatest need is often not for technical intervention, but for someone to talk to, and perceptive listening skills and appropriate guidance should be adequately rewarded.

Many physicians feel that the present system no longer satisfies the basic motivation that brought them into the health care field in the first place. They are also aware of the high divorce, bankruptcy, heart attack, and suicide rates among physicians and would appreciate a less stressful healthcare environment.

NURSES

I have known some fantastic nurses during my career. The ones that have left the strongest impression on me were not necessarily those with the best administrative skills. They were the ones who were truly 'there' for the patient, whether it meant holding the hand of an emotionally devastated soldier in VietNam who had had his legs blown off, or consoling a frightened child in my office. These nurses were also expert at subtly making suggestions for therapy that I may not have thought of, or quietly being supportive during crucial times in surgical procedures when nerves were frazzled and every moment counted.

Even excellent nurses sometimes buckle under the stress of hospital work. Much of the pressure seems unnecessary. A nurse's primary function is to enhance the healing of the patient. Real nursing is nurturing both for the patient and the nurse. However, nurses are often so busy attending to other things that at the end of the day they feel unfulfilled. These distractions include unreasonable demands by the patient for personal service unrelated to their illness, unreasonable criticism by impatient doctors, and administrative excesses by supervisors, whose focus is on having everything look good for the various peer review and quality assurance committees and governmental inspectors who are always looking over their shoulders. The order of priorities can sometimes become quite confusing.

Although the burnout rate for nurses is high in all departments, it is greatest in the most stressful units such as intensive care, surgery, and emergency rooms. This is not surprising, for death is often a visitor to these areas. Many nurses are unable to step back from their natural compassion and feel overly responsible, experiencing each death as a personal failure.

Ask any group of nurses, and you will find a deep undercurrent of discontent. The working hours are often disruptive of a normal family life because patients need nursing care 24 hours a day. Scheduling supervisors often do not (or cannot) take the personal needs of the nurse into consideration. Some other factors which nurses tell me contribute to their discontent are too much responsibility with too little respect, loss of direct patient contact, and loss of a feeling of being nourished on a personal level by the increasingly bottom-line oriented health institutions. Cold corporate mentality with its profit incentive have displaced a sense of community and of belonging in many hospitals.

Patients certainly sense all this confusion, discontent, and stress. Many wonder why the hospital is not a more pleasant and healing environment.

The Changing Concept of Disease

The origin of illness is being re-evaluated. Of course there are bacteria, viruses, and other known disease producing agents, but for many illnesses the cause is still unknown. No theory of the cause of illness seems to apply to all diseases. An illness often seems to happen to a person beyond his control and without his consent. On the other hand, there are cases when it is obvious that patients have participated in bringing on their ailments. Some examples are stress related heart disease, physical and emotional exhaustion making one more susceptible to a variety of illnesses, and cigarette smoking triggering lung cancer. Underlying this, however, is a deeper cause. Psychological emptiness may underlay the desire or need to smoke, to overeat, or to cause a person to push himself beyond healthy limits. A major part of this book will be taking a look at the psychological problems that underlie the more obvious external causes of disease.

In waging our war against disease over the past century or two, we have found wellness as elusive as a ghost, with various illnesses being vanquished but disease showing up in another form just when it seemed victory was near at hand.

Our efforts at identifying and eradicating the outside forces which we see as the perpetrators of diseases, though certainly helpful for some individual diseases, do not seem to be making much overall progress in eliminating disease as a whole. A plethora of new diseases has appeared. A few of these are AIDS, Alzheimer's Disease, Chronic Fatigue Syndrome, fibromyalgia, antibiotic resistant pneumonias, necrotizing skin infections, and increasing numbers of previously rare cancers and neurologic disorders.

There are toxins polluting the environment from overzealous use of insecticides, herbicides, and other synthetic chemicals. There is increasing radiation exposure from industrial and medical use of radioactive materials, continued nuclear weapon testing, and the unsolved problems of disposing of nuclear wastes. We have toxic mercury levels in our seafood, thinning of the ozone layer, and possible harmful low frequency waves from electrical sources. Many of these environmental poisons are demonstrating their effect on our immune systems and on our genes. Our health as well as the health of future generations is being jeopardized.

In addition, there are perhaps worse "diseases" taking a heavy toll. These have not previously been considered medical problems until they caused physical symptoms. They are the social diseases of poverty, ignorance, prejudice, isolation, and spiritual deprivation. They result in feelings of helplessness, hopelessness, frustration, confusion, anger, and inner conflict. This inner turbulence often manifests as addictions, school and social dropouts, street gangs, child and spousal abuse, felonies, killings, terrorists attacks, genocide, and even wars between nations.

How much evidence do we need before we can come to the conclusion that our search for the cause of disease has not been addressing the entire problem? At times it seems as though our health care leaders and health researchers are hidden away in ivory towers, diligently working in their laboratories on the minute details of various diseases, while we are literally drowning in a sea of suffering and chaos.

A Changing Medical Paradigm

NEW IDEAS, ALTERNATIVES

Startling new ideas are now being assimilated into Western thinking which questions the foundation of our concept of disease and medical care. Eastern healing philosophies, viewing disease as a form of disharmony at often invisible levels, use means for restoring harmony which often seem strange to our Western mentality. Long discounted by our scientifically oriented society, these theories and treatments are for the first time being given serious consideration by significant numbers of intelligent Westerners. Non-scientifically based remedies are not limited to Eastern traditions, and bookstores are filled with tantalizing, informative volumes about every alternative medical subject imaginable. Doctors are accustomed to informing patients about the latest medical technology and medications, but now patients also want to know about acupuncture, acupressure, aromatherapy, Aruvedic Medicine, bio-feedback,

Chinese herbal therapy, hypnotherapy, imagery, macrobiotic diets, massage therapy, meditation, past life regression, psychotherapy, spiritual healings, spontaneous remissions, subtle energy fields, therapeutic touch, and Yoga – to mention only a few. Looking at that list, it is obvious that many of these treatments are approaching healing from mental, emotional, and spiritual perspectives, rather than purely a physical one.

Patients who become discouraged because they are still suffering in spite of their present medical care, are anxious to reach for almost anything additional that offers hope. Many patients are no longer willing to accept morbid or hopeless prognoses from their physicians because they have come to believe that there are alternative treatments available. Also, patients are often hesitant to accept the physician's recommendations for massively invasive, and often very expensive, surgical procedures or medical treatments which are potentially life threatening or debilitating, without first investigating other options. The physician's undisputed authority as the only knowledgeable expert regarding the treatment of disease is being questioned. His role as the source of all healing has been undermined.

Many patients are already using alternative care modalities which most physicians consider unscientific, either in addition to or instead of, their usual, scientific (allopathic) medical care. In the frequently quoted study by David Eisenberg in the New England Journal of Medicine (Jan 28, 1995), it is estimated that over sixty million Americans annually use these 'nonscientific' treatments.[1] This must be a bit unsettling to a health care industry that has for years enjoyed a virtual monopoly. What may be even more threatening to the scientific medical establishment is that some of these patients who have jumped ship, so to speak, demonstrate improvement and even cures. There is an ongoing re-evaluation of the whole concept of just what is good medicine and what is bad medicine.

NEW QUANTUM THEORIES

Scientists are probing ever more deeply into the mysteries underlying not only illness, but life itself. Theories and discoveries in the nuclear age, especially the sub-atomic science of quantum physics, are remodeling our basic understanding of the nature of the universe. Our old comfortable Newtonian laws of physics, on which our allopathic medical system has been based, clearly separated the universe into the material world and the nonmaterial world. Since the latter could not be studied with scientific precision, it had long ago been discounted by the scientific community and had been left, uncontested, in the hands of philosophers and spiritual groups. It was felt this non-material (spiritual), non-physical (metaphysical) dimension was not involved in health and healing. Now it is beginning to appear this judgment was unsound.

The distinction that science had made between what it considered "real" and "unreal" has now been superseded by new scientific evidence that erases this previously distinct boundary. Theories in quantum physics, and the experimental observations supporting these theories, suggest a constantly changing reality, where the boundaries between various forms of matter and even the distinction between matter and energy are nonexistent.

Even more revolutionary, research at the quantum level of the particle-wave interface indicates that events can be influenced by intention or thought of the observer. In experiments to determine whether an electron is composed of matter or is pure energy, it was found that it could be either, depending on the answer that the experimenter wanted!

When one looks at the structure of an atom through the eyes and measurements of scientists, one sees tiny particles separated by giant spaces, much like the stars and planets with vast distances separating them. Add to this the idea that the particles are actually in constant motion, and at their most basic level are switching back and forth between being solid matter and wave-like energy. This gives us an entirely different way to see our bodies and everything else we have considered as solid matter. Instead of being something which our senses tell us is solid and stable, what we really are is mostly empty space, constantly in a state of change.

Now consider the possibility that our thoughts or intentions can influence the changes!

An example of this power of intention is the effect of meditation and intention on plant growth. In experimental studies, plants being "prayed for" grow faster and larger than others in similar environments which are not receiving these positive thoughts.[2] In other scientific studies, plants and animals can sense human emotions and are nurtured by a loving environment and stunted by a hostile environment.[3&4] On the level of human life, prayer has been shown to statistically improve the outcome of patients admitted to an intensive cardiac case unit.[5] Loving attention in many forms has been demonstrated to speed recovery.[6]

ENERGY FIELDS AND OTHER UNKNOWNS

This opens the door to new ideas, suggesting that forces outside the sphere of our current knowledge affect our material existence, and along with this, our health. Simply put, our thoughts and intentions activate some as yet unknown forces that can change our physical world, including our physical bodies.

What these forces or energy fields are remains unknown, but this does not mean they do not exist. Acupuncture is scientifically unexplained, but even the most skeptical materialist must be impressed when observing its remarkable effects. Unseen energy pathways apparently transmit effects to distant body areas.

Techniques of therapeutic touch such as Rieki and Jin Shin Jytsu, do have observable healing effects, possibly transmitting some type of energy, or changing energy fields through unseen pathways. As yet, I know of no scientific instruments able to accurately measure this energy or clearly demonstrate these pathways.

I recently had the opportunity to observe the effects of Jin Shin Jytsu.[7] Believe me, I am as skeptical about these strange treatments as anyone. A close personal friend was experiencing a very real problem with vertigo. His daily work activities involved climbing ladders and balancing in precarious positions, and he was completely disabled by this condition. He frequently became unbalanced and fell to one side when walking. His customary activity of tennis became impossible.

My friend went the usual scientific medical route, had numerous examinations by specialists in Internal Medicine, ENT, and Neurology. He had several studies including MRI. No specific cause for the vertigo was identified, and none of the prescribed treatments affected his vertigo at all. He also tried chiropractic therapy to no avail.

Noting his despair and having nothing else to offer, I casually suggested that he might contact a person I know who lives in his city, and is a practitioner and teacher of Jin Shin Jytsu. Even though this person had recounted to me some truly amazing anecdotal case histories, I had no idea that something so "unscientific" might have an effect on this disabling condition of vertigo, but thought it was worth a try.

After one treatment my friend says he was markedly improved, and after the second treatment his symptoms had subsided enough for him to resume working and playing tennis. He is definitely a convert, and I am not as skeptical as I once was!

One anecdotal case, unproven, one could say. There are simply too many similar case histories for me to continue to shut my eyes to such interesting treatment options. They may not always work wonders, but why not at least be open to giving them a fair trial? Different from many scientific medical treatments, they have no harmful side effects.

Hypnosis is another field which seems to be severely underutilized as a modality for diagnosis and treatment. The astounding powers of the mind under hypnosis have long been observed, many of which defy scientific explanation. I have been amazed at several cases where hypnotherapists have been able to bring about healing responses when other, more standard efforts had been unsuccessful. Their techniques of helping the patient explore the subconscious mind are gentle, nonthreatening, and depend on trust between the patient and therapist.

There are other historically recorded phenomena which demonstrate that the mind can control bodily responses, but since our society became so devoted to "pure" science, these truly remarkable observations have been ignored. There are Biblical examples of human beings being impervious to fire.

Also, there are similar, more recent, well documented, historical examples where numerous human beings were unable to be harmed by fire and other drastic punitive measures. These phenomena occurred during the persecution of the Huegenot religious sect in France and were observed by thousands of people and are well documented by the newspapers and other writings from that time. They are staggering in their implications.[8] In the present day, fire-walking ceremonies are an everyday observable occurrence in some other cultures. For the last few years, this same phenomenon is being experienced in the Western world by ordinary people who participate in seminars using fire-walking to demonstrate the power of the mind. These seminars culminate with the participants walking barefoot on burning coals, and those to whom I have talked did it successfully. Just how a body can do this without even making a blister has never been scientifically explained to my satisfaction.

Another fact that defies scientific reasoning is the 'placebo effect,' with 30% or even higher therapeutic response to chemically inert substitute medication.[9] The only logical explanation that makes sense to me is that if one believes, then the body responds according to those beliefs. In my own experience as a physician, I have seen healing responses which I am convinced occurred simply because the patient believed in the treatment.

There are too many fascinating case studies, and too many "miraculous" cures and other incongruences for which our hard scientific approach has no answers. I would suggest that for further inquiry and clear documentation of some of these truly astounding phenomena one should consult the amazing books, *A Holographic Universe,* by Dr. Michael Talbot, *Spontaneous Healing* by Andrew Weil, M.D., *The Future of the Body* by

Michael Murphy, and *Spontaneous Remission* by Brendon O'Regan and C. Hirchberg.[10]

DOCTOR'S DILEMMA

There seem to be no simplistic explanations anymore, and health care is being forced by a curious, informed, and demanding public to expand its boundaries into areas where issues and answers are not so black and white.

At times, medical doctors and other health professionals may find themselves feeling a bit unsettled with the implications of all this new information. They have given much of their lives to extensive and difficult scientific training and study, preparing for a position of authority and leadership in the health care field, and have fully expected to be honored and respected for their expertise. Instead, more and more often, their advice is being questioned, and patients are making decisions which the physician may feel are unwise. The doctor may see himself as being discounted by the very persons to whom he would be of service.

There seems to be a more ready admission among physicians today that perhaps scientific medicine just may not have all the answers, but there is uncertainty about where to turn for new direction. There are numerous possibilities out there that were not considered as treatment options during my medical training. For most of my medical career, I have valiantly defended scientific medicine and vigorously denied the validity of "alternative" medical treatments, but now I have expanded the limits of my acceptance and become more open-minded. Instead of feeling diminished by this broader concept, I feel encouraged that the field of healing is not as limited as I once thought.

One underlying fact seems consistent throughout: the ability to heal is an innate quality that resides within the patient. Research and experience are proving that this healing ability can be enhanced by various treatments at the physical and the nonphysical levels. There seems to be no limit to the possibilities, and perhaps one day things that now seem like miracles will be the expected outcome.

In this age of rapidly expanding knowledge and research in areas previously unexplored, I would be hesitant to tell any patient that a specific treatment is his only chance or last hope.

ALTERNATIVE PRACTITIONERS, GOVERNMENT AND POLITICS

How is all this new, non-scientific information affecting the medical scene? In the past, chiropractors, homeopaths, naturopaths, massage therapists, acupuncturists, hypnotherapists, and a lot of others in various "alternative" healing fields, were discounted and even ridiculed by medical doctors. When patients insisted on exploring alternative treatments, there was a smug feeling among the scientific health care community, and I certainly shared this feeling, which said: "OK, let the ignorant fools go and look somewhere else for their health care, but they will be back, because there is nothing else worthwhile out there!" I'm not so convinced anymore that these other modalities, which seem difficult to understand by the scientifically trained mind, are without healing value. I think many MDs today share my changing feelings.

Even if physicians do not accept alternative healing methods, they are feeling their effects economically and politically. A few years ago the alternative care providers were scattered and were not significant competitors in the larger game. Now they have collectively developed into a force which is competing in a very substantial way. Their views about medical care are being supported by more and more of the public, and their influence is being felt in the election of our legislators who make the laws regarding medical care and determine in large measure who gets paid, and in what amount.

There is no doubt that MDs have lost some of their power as the dominant force in the healing profession. But this change has not come about through no fault of their own. The medical profession must take its share of the blame. As pointed out to me by Dr. John O'Shaughnessey of Macon, Georgia, who is one of the most complete physicians that I know, we were given a sacred trust by our government to furnish medical care for the citizens. We were the only ones who could write prescriptions, admit patients to hospitals, and perform surgery. We were handed a virtual monopoly to oversee the nations health, and in many ways, we have failed in this responsibility.

We are guilty of inattention to some of the details of this trust. We failed to police our own ranks, making it necessary for us to be policed by the government and the insurance industry who pay for our mistakes. We also neglected a large part of our population. A system evolved under which too many sick people feel inadequately cared for. The public feels out of touch with doctors. Many feel the personal benefits of being a physician, which include wealth, power, prestige, and social status, are the primary motivating factors for medical doctors, these having replaced compassion and the desire to be a healing servant.

The public has become resentful. Whether this is justified or not is open to debate, but it seems the public is ready to rescind its mandate. Maybe this is not such a bad thing, for the task of being responsible for the health of the nation is more than can be borne by any mortal or group of mortals. I believe personal health is the primary responsibility of the individual, and the health of the nation will improve when more and more individuals assume this responsibility, and the medical profession can take its rightful role as advisor and assistant in the health and healing process.

Summary Of Medical System In Transition

There is certainly a pervasive climate of confusion and distrust within the whole arena of health care. Everyone has his own scapegoat to blame as the cause for the unfulfilled expectations, friction and inefficiency of the health care system. However, the present spectacle of patients, doctors, alternative care-givers, hospital administrators, health insurance carriers and government program directors pointing fingers and lambasting each other does not appear to be leading to any solutions. No one who is truly interested in healing enjoys seeing the medical care system functioning in this way.

CHAPTER 3

WHAT I DID NOT LEARN
IN MEDICAL SCHOOL

When I graduated from medical school my head was crammed full of facts but I felt completely inadequate at transferring this knowledge to treating patients. In my naive state of mind I was in awe of professors, department heads, staff members, and even residents only a year or more older than I was. They all seemed so knowledgeable, self-assured and straight thinking. I felt they knew all the answers and had raised them in my mind almost to a position of infallibility.

One can learn a lot by observing, and physicians happen to be in very choice seats. Every physician I know can tell amazing stories of very unusual experiences with patients, and the most impressive of these stories are ones where events did not go as expected. Swapping such stories is an entertaining pastime among physicians, but many seem hesitant to share these experiences publicly. Here are a few of my own learning experiences which convinced me that there was not always a logical scientific explanation.

Dead Or Alive?

A medical history interview with a patient when I was a first-year resident comes to mind. I asked if she was allergic to any medicines. She responded, "Yes! Absolutely do not give me any penicillin! The last time I was sick someone gave me a penicillin shot and I ended up in the morgue! Just before starting the embalming process the attendant noticed a faint movement of breathing and discovered I was still alive. They rushed me back to the hospital and I recovered." I was able to substantiate this incident in her medical records. Amazingly, all the scientific medical personnel and sophisticated equipment which pronounced her dead had been wrong!

Another unusual incident which I remember from my residency was the case of a male patient of approximately 60 years of age who underwent a radical retropubic prostatectomy (a major operation for the total removal of the prostate) for prostate cancer. The surgery was difficult, taking most of the morning. There was profuse bleeding during and following the surgical procedure which required numerous blood transfusions. By that evening the patient's condition had become critical. He suddenly went into cardiac arrest, with no blood pressure, no pulse and no respirations.

We sprung into action using every lifesaving procedure and medication available. His room immediately became crowded with doctors, nurses and resuscitative machines. Nothing was left undone, but after about 30 minutes, he showed no sign of responding. Examination by a cardiologist revealed "box caring" of the veins in the retina (the back of his eyeball), which was felt to be a sure sign that his blood had ceased to flow, and indicated that further efforts at resuscitation would be fruitless.

It was generally believed that after 10 or 15 minutes of

inadequate oxygen to the brain there would be irreversible damage, and logically we should stop resuscitative efforts. There was, however, still a very occasional faint electrical impulse on the EKG, so we did not stop our efforts. Quite amazingly the patient gradually began to respond. After another hour the life support machines were no longer necessary. He soon regained consciousness and eventually recovered. There was no evidence of brain damage.

My sense of awe regarding the infallibility of scientific medicine began to crack a bit. If it was possible that well-trained medical practitioners could be mistaken about something as basic as judging whether a person was alive or dead, maybe they were as human and prone to mistakes as the rest of us.

Unpredictable Outcome

Other experiences taught me that individuals were different in their response to treatment. For example, two persons may have the same illness and receive the same treatment. One recovers, the other dies. I noticed that outward physical appearance and apparent stability are not always reliable in predicting one's health. A person who outwardly demonstrates the picture of perfect health may have a sudden severe myocardial infarction or develop a rapidly fatal malignancy. On the other hand, someone who appears terribly unhealthy and has the most destructive life habits may continue to indulge himself, and mock everyone's warnings and predictions of disaster by surviving for years. Patients appearing to be healthy can die suddenly of unexpected post-operative complications. Others who appear to be near-impossible risks go through massive surgery and recovery without suffering any complications. All of these observations gradually led me to the conclusion that my training and understanding about the cause and treatment of physical illness did not take into account other mysterious factors that were important.

Uncertain Cause

I recall an acquaintance who, at age 32, had a sudden severe coronary artery occlusion, or in layman's terms, a massive heart attack. His testimony was that he was well and feeling fine until this happened. Now he was disabled and angry, and he blamed fate for inflicting this condition upon him and ruining his life. His close friends saw the situation differently. They gave the following interpretation of the event: "We could see this coming on. He was under a lot of pressure in his job, his family life was in trouble. He was anxious and worried all the time, though he tried not to show it. We were not surprised when we heard the news." Several questions remained unanswered: When did this man's illness begin? Where was the origin of his illness? Did it originate in his coronary arteries or was the original focus of the disease in his mind? Could there be some connection between his thoughts, his fears and other emotions, and the physical manifestation of his disease? His friends seemed to think so.

My 1960s medical training would tell me his illness was possibly of genetic origin. Outside of that, I recall no other offered explanation, and heart attacks seemed to happen purely by chance. Later, diet began to be viewed as important, and jogging became popular, so the 1980s and 1990s view might be that he probably ate too much fatty food and did not exercise enough, and if he had watched his cholesterol levels more closely this could have been avoided.

People who do all these things still have heart attacks. I can no longer accept any of these explanations as completely adequate. It seems more reasonable to me to believe that mental attitude does have a direct affect on the physical health of our bodies, including the coronary arteries. It is becoming evident that mental factors, at the least contribute to, and possibly are the primary cause of, many cases of coronary artery occlusion as well as many other diseases.

No Guarantee

Another example from my practice that caused me to question my concept of disease and its proper treatment was a patient, and friend, who came to see me because she had noticed a small amount of blood in her urine. Mrs. B. was an exceptionally delightful person. She was approximately 55 years old, lived with a loving husband and was close to a very supportive family. Together they owned and operated a plant nursery and were very much an active part of our small community.

Prompt investigation revealed a kidney cancer. She underwent a surgical procedure to remove this kidney and the surrounding tissue. Her recovery was uneventful, and tests revealed that the malignancy was confined to the kidney with no evidence of spread to other parts of her body. Her prognosis was excellent.

Mrs. B. returned to a full and robust life. I looked forward to seeing her for her semi-annual checkups. Her case was an affirmation of the correct doctor-patient relationship as I had been taught to understand it: The patient is to be alert for early symptoms, report them promptly to the physician, follow his expert advice, and be assured that everything will be fine. What a nice easy formula for perfect health and long life! Too bad it doesn't always work!

Approximately six or seven years after her surgery, her routine chest x-ray showed multiple metastatic nodules which proved to be the same cancer which had originated in the kidney. No treatment was effective. She died within six months.

The seeds of this kidney cancer, living cancer cells, had obviously been present in her body all along, but remained dormant until inexplicably something about her physiology changed. I have no clue as to what might have happened to make her immune system ineffective after six years of successfully holding her cancer in abeyance.

This case, and others like it, began to open my mind to doubt about the veracity of what I was believing and telling patients. It was disheartening to see that even when everyone played the game strictly by the rules the outcome was still uncertain. It seemed there was something very important that we were missing.

At that time, the concept of the immune system as a key element in the body's defense mechanism was not widely understood. The primary focus of cancer treatment was on early diagnosis and prompt radical treatment. On reading the current medical literature and noting the present day advice of the American Cancer Society, I am impressed that this focus has not changed much even today. In spite of a significant broadening of the understanding of the importance of the immune system and how it can be enhanced or depressed, this information does not appear to be a part of most treatment planning.

There is more interest now on enhancing the effectiveness of the immune system through modifications in diet and physical activity, and in lifestyle changes. There is less open, but increasing, acceptance of the idea that the mind and attitude also influence the immune system. It is well established fact that potentially life-threatening cancer cells commonly occur in everyone, but that our immune systems recognize these abnormal cells and destroy them. No one has as yet discovered what factor, or combination of factors, disrupts this immune system function and allows these malignant cells to survive and continue to grow and multiply, eventually resulting in clinical cancer.

Is Illness A Choice?

Other cases were many equally perplexing, but for different reasons. One kind and loving patient was ill and bedridden for at least 30 years, only arising for funerals and weddings and other special events, but always looking splendid at these occasions. As I remember, she was a mild diabetic and she also took medicine for some type of heart problem. She appeared well enough to be more actively participating in life, but by her own wishes she stayed confined, being cared for by her immediate family. She corresponded frequently and eloquently with a large number of relatives and friends. When visited she was actively interested and enthusiastic about everyone's lives and activities. For her own unshared and probably unknown reasons, she had chosen to be content to be an observer of life rather than an active participant. She must have had an emotional need for a role that required her to remain confined and to appear helpless, and wellness was somehow unacceptable to her. She eventually quietly passed away, but not until she had attained the ripe old age of 88.

I had several patients who absolutely refused to stay well. When cured of one physical problem, they would rapidly develop another. Treating them was somewhat like joining with them in the childhood game of "hide and seek" where when one hiding place is discovered, a new game begins and the child must find a new place to hide. It would have been easy to discount these patients as being overly imaginative, except that the diseases often proved to be real and were confirmed on physical exam and laboratory and x-ray studies. This "game" continued until finally the individual would come up with something that was incurable. At this point, I could almost detect a sigh of relief, or an unspoken message like "I won! I was right all along. I knew I was really sick and nobody would believe me." Lord knows what mental abberations these diseases were hiding.

Am I Really Listening?

There seem to be innumerable lessons to learn, and each person we meet has the potential for being our teacher. One of my best teachers, although he probably doesn't know it, was a patient I saw several years ago in Mississippi. His presenting problem of mild urinary symptoms quite reasonably caused him to be concerned about his prostate. His evaluation required three or four office visits.

This patient was a medical practitioner and was quite personable and we chatted at length. He was probably 55, or about 10 years older than I was at the time. He was handsome, well groomed, in excellent physical condition and appeared at the peak of success in all areas of his life. He had successfully raised several children to maturity, had a stable and loving marriage and a fine medical practice. He owned a beautiful home, a second seashore vacation home, several expensive automobiles, club memberships, and a yacht.

I admit that at the time, I was a little envious of his material success, but I was also inspired. I felt my goals were quite similar to what he had achieved, and I was on the right track. If I could just keep plugging along, keep my "nose to the grindstone," I was thinking, then I could eventually be equally successful, and therefore happy and contented with my life.

At his last office visit, after assuring him that I had found no problem or cause for concern regarding his prostate, I confided to him my admiration and envy of what he had made of his life and my desire to emulate it. He became quiet and rather thoughtful for a moment and appeared a bit perplexed. I was totally shocked when he then said, "It seems I did not tell you the whole story. The truth is, I have been so unhappy and depressed lately that I have been seriously considering suicide!"

From a medical perspective I certainly learned from this gentleman that you cannot always "judge a book by its cover,"and that the state of a person's health is more than just physical appearance. I had never really considered what might be going on in this patient's mind, because, like most of us, he was an expert in covering up his true feelings. I was so focused on his presenting complaint, and saw only his external mask of health and apparent happiness, that I never considered looking deeper.

He did not commit suicide, and I hope he was able to resolve his problems before they manifested in emotional breakdown or physical disease. I have since tried to be more perceptive to what is going on below the surface of the presenting complaint.

There Must Be More Than This

At the time, I was becoming discontented and feeling somewhat inadequate with medical practice as I was experiencing it. It had begun to dawn on me that in treating only the physical disease, I may be only treating the physical manifestation of some illness which was in truth originating on a much deeper level. Since everyone's body eventually dies, if my treatment was aimed solely at cure of physical disease, then I was doomed to a 100% failure rate. This was particularly distressing to me, as I was practicing in a small community where most of the patients were friends, and many were relatives, and I was now often seeing the terminal stages of their diseases.

From another, more personal perspective, the encounter with the above described depressed and suicidal patient was very important to me. I began to look differently at my life, my goals, and my activities. I realized that I was not really living! I was constantly sacrificing my ability to be happy and joyful in the present moment for some future rosy dream when I would be free of responsibilities and would have the time and the money to do the things I really enjoyed. As I recall, this is about the time when my personal mid-life crisis began. That could be a chapter with which many would identify. My particular version of this life passage included all the emotional devastation (and also the opportunity for growth) of finally admitting to being completely confused and discontented with life as I had been experiencing it. Although I was not physically ill, I knew that my life was out of balance, and just admitting to myself there was a problem allowed me to start looking for answers.

CHAPTER 4

PERSONAL SPIRITUAL REFORMATION

The preceding paragraphs perhaps explain how I became interested in looking for other explanations of disease. I also felt unhealed myself. There was an emptiness inside which was telling me something else was desperately needed for my personal growth.

I did not understand it at the time, but now believe any valid concept of healing must contain a spiritual element. Until a few years ago, my own sense of spirituality was very confused and underdeveloped. Although there was no conscious planning, the Universe seemed to direct some changes in my core spiritual concepts.

Early Training:
Fear And Unworthiness

For years I had indulged in sporadic, half-hearted attempts to find an inner spiritual truth that would allow me to feel some inner assurance that I was at least on the right track toward some higher goal, call it Salvation, the Kingdom of Heaven, or just plain peace, happiness, and contentment. Raised a Catholic and later an Episcopalian, I was a "believer" in some mysterious all-powerful God, and I had an acceptance of Jesus Christ as an example of the way to peace and to "Heaven," but my actions belied the fact that I had no deep conviction of just what this all meant. The Bible, which to me is a wonderful source of inspiration, also seemed to contain many conflicting messages. So many questions remained unanswered. The answers offered by the religious traditions with which I was acquainted seemed contradictory, incomplete, or even at times nonsensical.

I am thankful for my upbringing in the Roman Catholic church, which incorporated some truly rich, life-affirming traditions into my belief system, but I regret that there were many notions implanted that I now believe were harmful and severely limiting to my personal spiritual growth. These notions definitely interfered with my ability to find inner harmony and self acceptance. Let me try to clarify.

I was taught to be God-fearing. I was convinced that I was essentially a "bad" person and that only by sacrifice and continuous striving could I hope to be worthy; and only by waging an unending fight against my animal instincts could I ever win my way into God's favor and have any hope for His approval and acceptance at some final terrifying Last Judgment. To be perfectly honest, I wasn't very good at sacrifice and endless striving, and my animal instincts were quite strong. At times I was consumed by guilt, and I felt hopelessly doomed.

Thankfully, there was another teaching within the same religious tradition that saw God as loving and forgiving. This did not seem compatible with a stern, judgmental, punishing God. I did not know how to reconcile these two conflicting ideologies, but I knew that the forgiving philosophy was my only hope, so I begged for mercy in my prayers.

Jesus Christ was supposed to be my example and model for the ideal pathway to the heart of God, but I was disheartened because he was so perfect and never made a mistake. As hard as I might try to demonstrate his admirable qualities outwardly, in the hidden recesses of my mind, I saw myself as a miserable failure. Guilt and shame became my internal companions. Mea culpa! Mea culpa! Mea maxima culpa! (I am guilty! I am guilty! I am most guilty!) was the message I had absorbed from my church. Even today, I tend to revert back to this self-defeating internal criticism if I am not mindful.

Gradual Change

I do not think that I could have ever been willing to probe into this area had I stuck with a "cut and dried" religious belief system that allowed little room for questioning dogma. For many years I had remained an active member of the church, Catholic and later Episcopal. I believed that close identification with some organized religion was a requirement to spiritual comfort.

I clearly remember an incident which happened shortly after I had joined Kathy in attending the small Episcopal Church in Brookhaven, Mississippi. We would join others for lessons and discussion after the Sunday church service. One Sunday as I was half listening and half looking around, my attention became focused on a poster in the corner of the room. Its message was, "Christ came to win your heart, not to control your mind." I liked that, and felt I had found a new spiritual home.

I eventually had to give up identifying myself with either church, however, as I realized that parts of each belief system were incompatible with my reason and heartfelt sense of truth. I became rather cynical about any "belief system," and was later amused. and somewhat in agreement with, Robert Monroe's observation, (which I heard at the Monroe Institute in Faber, Virginia,) that he thought it was no accident that these two words could be shortened to "BS."

Loren's Death

My personal spiritual developmental retardation was brought into intense focus on the evening of January 7, 1989, with the sudden accidental death of my beloved stepdaughter, Loren Quinn. I was driving our family home from a movie one night when suddenly our mini-van was slammed into and overturned by a sports car driven by a drag-racing teenager. Loren was thrown out and crushed beneath our Nissan mini-van. Kathy and Rafe and I were all unhurt. I tried desperately to resuscitate Loren for what seemed like an eternity as I felt her life slipping away. The emergency technicians arrived and took over, but all to no avail. She never regained consciousness and was pronounced dead on arrival at the hospital.

It was as though a bolt of lightning had come out of the blue, taking Loren away and changing our lives forever. Nothing in my belief system could offer any reasonable explanation for the seemingly random, senseless loss of this beautiful, joyful child, just at the threshold of a life that appeared to hold forth unlimited potential.

My wife, Kathy, was even more devastated than I, but she reminded me of Jacqueline Kennedy as she somehow maintained her composure and managed to suppress her grief and make the difficult decisions required during those first few days. Her calmness was an emotional lifesaver for me and many others who were grieving. Later, her graceful forgiveness and extension of friendship to the young man who had caused the accident were remarkable and inspirational. Her grieving for Loren has been slow and long, and still surfaces at times. Thanks to the efforts of so many friends, family, new acquaintances, accidental discoveries, prayers, letters, and shoulders to cry on, we gradually began to heal.

Accelerated Change

Kathy was determined to know more about the afterlife and wanted desperately to understand what had happened to her dear lost child. We embarked on an intensive spiritual search. Unlike me, Kathy did not recognize any restrictions and was not bound by any deeply ingrained dogmatic beliefs. In my anger and grief, I was able to cast aside my own confining ideology.

To our joyful surprise, we discovered a vast array of spiritual information previously unknown to us. This great wealth of material is the result of man's eternal quest to discover the true nature of his Reality. It astounded me that the thoughts and words of so many brilliant enlightened beings is available to anyone who is willing to search. Only my narrow-mindedness had blinded me to the existence of a library of information far greater than I had ever imagined.

When The Student Is Ready
The Teacher Will Appear

I must recount an enlightening, and now rather amusing, incident that occurred shortly after Loren's death. Kathy received a very heart-warming letter from a stranger and she responded, first by calling this lady and then visiting her. As was later explained to Kathy by this newfound friend, the letter was the result of this lady's "inner guidance" which had repeatedly prompted her to write. She resisted until finally the letter was presented to her mind in completed form, and she could no longer ignore the urging. In spite of her fears of appearing "weird" to someone she did not know, she completed and sent the letter.

Kathy was inspired by this letter, and delighted with her new friend, who gave her hope regarding the eternal nature of Loren's soul and the possibility that their separation was only temporary. Kathy was happy to have a confidant who was open and accepting, and with whom she could discuss her feelings. The lady was a member of a Spiritualist church, and had a regular weekly meditation group that met at her home. Kathy was invited to attend this group.

I was suspicious of this unknown thing called meditation, and was also quite concerned from a medical standpoint about the state of Kathy's mental health. She had become more and more withdrawn and depressed since the accident. However, when she came home from this first meditation experience, she was exhilarated. She told me several of the ladies had "seen and received a message from Loren." This was completely outside the boundaries of what I understood at the time as normal behavior, and I was certain I would be forced to commit Kathy for psychiatric care!

Fortunately I did nothing, and over the next few months my opposition toward the mysterious softened and I also developed a openness to new possibilities. The Universe seemed to cooperate as I removed my blinders. I found new meaning in the injunction of Jesus Christ: "Seek and you shall find, Knock and the door will be opened unto you." Other passages in the Bible began to make more sense to me. I also found messages of hope and encouragement in nature, songs, poems, on billboards, and in everyday experiences.

Building Blocks Of Faith

One of the hymns sung at Loren's funeral was "I Will Bear You Up On Eagle's Wings." Afterwards, I began to take particular notice of the presence of eagles, which are plentiful in Central Florida. One of the first mornings I returned to work after Loren's death, I sighted an eagle flying overhead, seemingly leading my car, right above the highway. A few weeks later, we were spending the weekend at a second home we owned in St. Cloud, Florida, on the shore of a large lake. Kathy was sunbathing in the yard, I was sitting on a point of land about 150 yards away, and Rafe was in a power boat with a friend quite a distance out into the lake. A beautiful, white-headed bald eagle flew overhead, circled low and almost landed on the ground in front of me. He then flew directly toward the house and circled over Kathy. I watched almost entranced as he then flew to where Rafe was in the boat and circled over him, this time spiraling higher and higher until he disappeared from sight.

This unusual behavior of the eagle was a very affirming spiritual experience for me. I felt that in some way this eagle represented Loren. I sensed she was telling us she was all right, was present and alive, and was looking over us.

On another occasion, I was meditating before going to sleep, and was apparently in that twilight zone between sleep and wakefulness when suddenly, I experienced the most vivid and thrilling sensation, like flying through the air, and could even feel the wind blowing my hair. I felt vibrantly awake and tried to call out to Kathy who was in another room, but no sound would come out. I experienced a sensation of the mattress moving, as though someone was lying down beside me. I became very quiet and still and then felt an arm gently embracing me over my abdomen. I strongly sensed this was Loren, and was afraid to move lest she go away. To reassure myself I was not just imagining this, I reached up and placed my hand on this arm, and stroked it and felt the hand and the unmistakable long slender fingers that were Loren's. I never saw anything with my eyes, and this sensory apparition gradually faded. I was completely shaken and in tears, but filled with wonder and joy at the experience.

This experience was especially meaningful to me. Loren was my step-daughter. When Kathy and I married, I am sure I was considered an intruder. Her dream, I believe, was that her father and mother would make up and get back together. She loved her father dearly and spent much of her time with him, but tragically, 13 months after Kathy and I were married he suffered a severe heart attack and died at the young age of 37.

After that Loren and I got along well enough, and I am sure she appreciated me, but she could never be loving and cuddly like a natural child. She kept her safe distance, treated me with respect, but would always turn her cheek when we kissed. The beautiful experience after her death of being hugged by her from another realm was so wonderfully affirming that I came away from it knowing she had forgiven me. I was convinced she did love me, and had given up her misperception that I had somehow tried to displace her father.

Kathy and Rafe, and even our housekeeper had some similar experiences. Kathy's most dramatic "visitation" occurred one evening while she was quietly alone on the couch, not really thinking about Loren or trying in any way to contact her. Suddenly Loren appeared, sitting in front of her on another part of the L-shaped couch. She looked well and happy, was dressed in shorts, sitting with her legs crossed and swinging her foot. She appeared almost solid, but not quite. Kathy received the very clear telepathic message: "Mom! When are you going to get it that I am all right!"

The beautiful vision was interrupted by the ringing of the telephone. Quite agitated, Kathy picked up the receiver and spat out "Hello!" Much to her amazement she was informed by the gentle voice of the caller that a location for the newly founded Loren Quinn Institute had been found.

I have not completely healed from the hurt and grief of our loss of Loren, but I can now truly thank her for being my wake-up call. (What a shame that I had missed so many earlier opportunities to begin opening my spiritual eyes!) Loren's death was the catalyst that brought about my personal "born again" experience, which I see as a shift in focus from the ephemeral to the eternal. Before, I had concentrated my time and attention on trying to make sense of the material world and on making my life experience more pleasurable. Now, however, I began to see the world through different eyes.

An example of how much easier it is to receive messages with a more open and willing mind happened to me in a very unlikely place, the St. Cloud, Florida, flea market! I was deep in the grieving process, very confused and unhappy, just trying to cope on a day-to-day basis, when I wandered into a booth where old books were being sold. A copy of *The Lives Of The Saints* caught my eye, and I casually flipped it open. In the middle of the opened page was a short paragraph describing a saint whose name I do not remember. It only said something to the effect that "This saint was called the Happy Saint. When asked why he was always so happy, he replied: 'No matter what happens to me, I know that nothing can ever take my God away from me.'"

Those words at another time might have had no effect on me, but during that time of despair, they were exactly what I needed to hear. I had probably been exposed to that same idea many times in various doctrines, but it had never taken root. Apparently the soil had not been fertile in the past, but now the message struck home. Deep within my soul some chord of ancient wisdom began to vibrate. I felt a shift within the core of my belief system. My despair lifted and I wanted to shout with joy. Although I still could not fully comprehend the day-to-day tragedies of this confusing world, I did now have an internal knowing that the God of my understanding does care for me and will not leave me. I understood for the first time that my true happiness and sense of well-being and worthiness does not depend on anyone or anything "out there," but is based purely upon an internal awareness of this relationship between the loving Creator and myself. There was no longer any reason for anything or anybody, even death of the body, to make me unhappy, unless I forgot and allowed it.

We were attending the Episcopal Church of the Good Shepherd, and I began to pay more attention to our minister's messages. At the time, fundamentalist groups and individuals were widely predicting the eminent "Second Coming" of Christ, and our minister interrupted his regular sermon to comment on the public fascination about this issue. He said the thing that bothered him most about the predictions was they implied that Christ was not with us at the present. "If you want to see the Christ," he said, "then turn and look at the person sitting next to you." I was stunned by the idea! But when I did what he asked and looked around at the others in the church, I saw a holiness in them that I had never seen before. Although I did not see a supernatural Being, I had an inner knowing that he had spoken a Truth. Could it be possible, I asked myself, that the Christ is in me and in everyone else?

These spiritual experiences and wonderful new concepts became like building blocks of faith for me. They seemed to be making their way into my awareness through some Graceful energy beyond my own will, but which simply felt right. And most of all, they made me long for more.

A Course In Miracles

I received another profound gift of Grace when I discovered a book called *A Course in Miracles*.[1] Kathy had purchased this book, and I was attracted by the title. When I picked it up and read the preface, all the fears of my early religious upbringing jumped up! Here, it seemed, was a 'channeled' book which gave evidence of having been dictated by the living Spirit of Jesus Christ! The material was compiled by two prominent psychologists from Columbia University, but they claimed no authorship, expressing only that the information had been written down precisely as instructed, by an Inner Voice which identified itself as Jesus Christ.

At that time, I had never heard of any such thing. I believed that the words of Jesus had been recorded in the Bible, and that was that! Whatever one needed to know for salvation was recorded there, and one simply needed to interpret it properly to find all the answers. Of course, in the same Bible, Jesus tells us that he will be with us always, but I believed this to be merely a figurative promise, not a literal one. I thought it could not be possible for Jesus to actually communicate with people and have them write down his message for others to see.

About two days after I had fearfully put this book aside, I received an unsolicited book in the mail from Loren's uncle, whom I hardly knew. It was *Journey Without Distance*,[2] and it described in detail all the circumstances involved in the transcribing and publication of A *Course in Miracles*. After reading this, I picked up A *Course in Miracles* again, and hardly put it down for the next six months.

The study of this material resonated so forcefully within me, and still does, that I felt the entirety of my life had been building up to the discovery of this information. It was an experience of joyfully being swept up and elevated to a new plain of awareness. I have heard others talk of their personal transformational experiences, and this, I believe, was mine. It was not a matter of this book instead of the Bible, but Jesus' message of love and forgiveness came through to me in modern terminology and psychological language that I could understand. His message 2000 years ago, for his audience at that time, was perfect in its imagery of grape vines, fig trees, loaves and fishes. It seemed to me, he was clarifying his message now for 20th century mankind.

I was so excited about this book I made a nuisance of myself. I gave it to my friends and relatives, and couldn't for the life of me understand why all of them were not equally impressed. It took me awhile to recognize that everyone was on his or her own chosen path, and that it was not up to me to change anyone. My job was my own healing and inner peace. A *Course in Miracles* (ACIM) certainly does not claim to be for everybody, and while the book allows that it is one course, it does not by any means claim to be the only course. I knew, however, that it was my course.

Fortunately, Kathy also became inspired to study, digest, and accept the validity of this material. Although we have not limited our search for truth to this one source, for me it has been a sounding board, a method by which I have been able to discover common universal gems of wisdom in many spiritual philosophies. I feel so fortunate to have a life companion with whom to share this spiritual journey, and Kathy and I have many lively conversations in which we vigorously test our new found concepts and try to apply them to life situations. As we studied ACIM, we discovered others who were also learning this material, and joined with groups who helped us understand.

Birds Of A Feather

There seems to be a universal law of magnetism that brings persons of similar interests together. Maybe this is not so profound, since it is known that "birds of a feather flock together." In fact, one of them practically landed on our doorstep when Carol Howe moved into our community. She flew here from Denver, Colorado, and stayed at our home while she looked for her new residence. She is a most enlightened teacher of the spiritual principles of A *Course in Miracles*, and specializes in their psychological application through lectures and workshops, and also through her writing.[3]

Our circle of friends rapidly expanded to include others who were similarly interested in trying to discover some truth that would give a higher meaning to their lives. Many of them had been through life-changing experiences which had forced them out of complacency. For some, it was a personal loss such as ours. For others, it was another challenge such as loss of a relationship, financial collapse, or the discovery of a life-threatening medical problem. There are also some who demonstrate that it is possible to 'wake up' without major trauma, but few, I think, can do it that way.

Attitudinal Healing

We met Dr. Jerry Jampolsky, the founder of the concept of Attitudinal Healing, at a seminar in Naples, Florida, and later attended a workshop at his original Attitudinal Healing Center in Tiburon, California.[4] He and his wife, Diane Cirincione, through their many inspirational books and their personal assistance, helped us open our own center, the Loren Quinn Institute for Attitudinal Healing.

Through the combined efforts of many of our wonderful, exciting new friends, the Loren Quinn Institute (LQI) came into being. The LQI was an Attitudinal Healing Center, where the outreach consisted of free support groups serving individuals going through all types of personal traumatic situations or illnesses, as well as those who simply needed a forum to express problems and be listened to in an accepting, nonjudgemental, unconditionally loving way. We all envisioned the Loren Quinn Institute as a safe place where anyone would be welcome, could feel free to discuss his or her own frustrations with life, and also explore ideas for mental, emotional, and spiritual enrichment and healing. Our involvement with the Loren

Quinn Institute, and now also with the Network for Attitudinal Healing International, Inc.[5] has rewarded us a hundred fold. The philosophy of Attitudinal Healing, which is basically that you can *change your life by changing your mind*, continues to be a guiding force and challenge toward healing ourselves. Health, in the principles of Attitudinal Healing, is defined as Inner Peace.

Although the Loren Quinn Institute no longer exists as a physical entity, there are still local groups using the Principles of Attitudinal Healing and the techniques of empathic listening. Many of those who were exposed to the groups and workshops at the LQI continue to use this newfound knowledge in their relationships, workplaces, support groups, church circles, etc., and have found an inner peace in their lives that was not possible for them in the past.

The Twelve Principles of Attitudinal Healing

1. *The essence of our being is love.*

2. *Health is inner peace. Healing is letting go of fear.*

3. *Giving and receiving are the same.*

4. *We can let go of the past and of the future.*

5. *Now is the only time there is and each instant is for giving.*

6. *We can learn to love ourselves and others by forgiving rather than judging.*

7. *We can become love-finders rather than fault-finders.*

8. *We can choose and direct ourselves to be peaceful inside regardless of what is happening outside.*

9. *We are students and teachers to each other.*

10. *We can focus on the whole of life rather than the fragments.*

11. *Since love is eternal, death need not be viewed as fearful.*

12. *We can always perceive ourselves and others as either extending love or giving a call for love.*

Further Discoveries

As our search continued, Kathy and I discovered the Monroe Institute[6] in Faber, Virginia, where we began to appreciate some understanding of the power of the mind and of meditation. We each had significant inner experiences there which were very powerful and clarifying for us.

We sought out lectures and workshops, read books, listened to tapes, watched videos, and in these ways became acquainted with inspirational thinkers, speakers and writers from many spiritual traditions. Through seminars, study groups, and religious services, we found new friends who were loving, accepting, and open to new ideas. It was invigorating to discover a freshness and inquisitiveness about spirituality which we had not experienced before.

Emphasis On Healing

Through our efforts and willingness to be open to new ideas and experiences, we could feel ourselves healing from the wounds of life. In all of the spiritual material we were studying, there was an underlying focus on healing. Spiritual wholeness came to mean an intrinsic state of peaceful existence and seemed to be a vital ingredient of 'healthy' people. These were often not wealthy or particularly successful by worldly standards, but they exuded a warmth which was magnetic, which seemed to come from a knowing inside that they were OK. They may not even be physically well, and frequently showed the damaging effects of disease, but this only made their qualities of inner peace more impressive. They appeared to have an inextinguishable joy that was not affected by the trials and tribulations of life.

Health or wellness seemed to be a more wholesome and peaceful sense of belonging to some greater reality which was not visible, and was therefore metaphysical or within the realm of spirit. The outer appearance of a healthy body or worldly success could be present in anyone, but it was often the loss of these outer trappings which revealed the true state of spiritual health of the individual.

My mind was literally being retrained to think differently about the subject of healing. For nearly thirty years, I had been focused on medical treatment of the body, and to a lesser extent of the mind. Now, I was finally working on the third part, the spiritual aspect, of a more holistic view of healing. Entirely new concepts regarding health, and healing, disease began to take shape in my mind.

CHAPTER 5

REDEFINING HEALTH, HEALING, AND DISEASE

This book is not about a right or a wrong way of seeing and doing things. I am not supporting any cause, or crusading for physicians to move to a more holistic view of medicine. However, life has more meaning when viewed through a wider angle lens, and this change to a broader view is occurring.

I have had my own struggles in breaking through my scientifically trained mind-set to a position of being able to accept there is healing to be found through many disciplines. It has taken a lot of time and many patients for me to learn scientific medicine does not have all the answers. Now, I must admit I have observed some very healthy responses in people taking alternative treatments which sound bizarre or absurd.

After deciding to put my judgement aside, I have become a friend and admirer of many alternative practitioners, and find most are not charlatans, as I once believed, but are sincere in their quest for healing, and no more motivated by the desire for monetary reward than scientific medical professionals. I have decided it is not my responsibility to judge or be critical of what a person chooses as his or her pathway for healing.

It is time to end the war of words and criticism between the scientific health care community and the alternative care-givers, because it is unworthy of either and demeaning to both. There is common ground on which everyone interested in healing can stand and share and be counted. Our goal can be to emphasize our common quest for healing rather than continuing to argue about our conflicting opinions.

If we are to become less rigid, if we are to be willing to expand our concept of health and healing, then the least threatening and most logical place to start may be at the very bottom. By that I mean at the level of definitions and core beliefs about health, healing, and disease. The place to begin re-evaluating and restructuring our concepts about the health care system is at its foundation.

Definition Of Health

Perhaps we can come to agreement on a definition of health that is much broader than the one commonly in use today. The American Heritage Dictionary defines health as, "The state of an organism functioning normally without disease or abnormality." It is hard to improve on that definition. However, it depends entirely on one's concept of disease or abnormality. Most of us are working from a limiting perspective of disease which has considered only the physical body as the diseased part of the organism. It is time to expand our limited concept of health to include the wholeness of the body, the mind, and the spirit.

Although healing has customarily been thought of as physical recovery from a bodily disease or injury, surely there are also deep wounds in our emotional, mental, and spiritual realms which require healing as well.

Defining <u>HEALTH</u> as: *"Optimal harmonious functioning of an individual on all levels of body, mind, and spirit,"* is better, but still is not enough. Any individual unable to have a successful relationship, or possessing an undying hatred of others, or threatening the health of our environment cannot be considered entirely healthy either. Realizing that our individual health depends on our connectedness with each other and with all that is, I would add to our original definition: *"and effective, life-enhancing interrelationships between oneself and other individuals, society, and nature."*

Definition Of Healing

When thinking about healing, we need to consider its source. As a person heals, he may be assisted by a physician, a nurse, alternative health care-givers, or medical treatments, but the healing actually comes from within.

As a physician, I have become convinced of the importance of a desire to heal within the mind of the patient, to bring about a healing bodily response. Unless he/she makes a decision from a dominant part of the will (conscious or subconscious) to be alive and well, no amount of outside support or treatment will be effective for long.

It may not be possible to determine from one's outward behavior or affect whether he/she truly desires healing or not. Often the desire to heal and to live may be present on one level of consciousness, but this conflicts with the opposite desire on another level. Some may outwardly profess a desire to get well, but emotionally have already given up hope. We have all seen this in patients afflicted with a serious illness who only feign putting up a fight. Other patients are in so much physical or emotional pain that they outwardly express a desire to die, but even in situations of the worse suffering, there may still exist a strong will to live below the level of conscious awareness.

A dramatic movie scene from *The Exorcist* demonstrates this latter point. I generally disagreed with the concept of this movie because it presented the idea that outside forces control us against our will. However, in one particular scene, the pathetic, "possessed" young girl was displaying her most abominable, despicable behavior and her priest-healer was about to become discouraged. She had to be sedated heavily to make her rest, and while she was sleeping, from somewhere deep within her subconscious the message "HELP" arose and appeared as dermatographic writing on the skin of her chest. Obviously, the patient still harbored a deep desire to heal and to live. Though fictional, this scene dramatically displays that often we do not understand a person's internal motivations.

Further emphasizing that often it is not obvious where the impetus for healing comes from, is an amazing story related to me by a friend whom I met at the annual convention of the National Institute for the Clinical Application of Behavioral Medicine in Orlando in 1991. She is a trained nutritionist and mental health counselor, and in addition has spent several years in China learning herbal therapy and an Eastern technique of healing touch.

She has a private counseling practice, and had been consulted by the parents of a six-month old daughter who was dying of AIDS. The child had contracted this disease from a life-saving blood transfusion from her father after a severe auto accident had ruptured her liver and spleen. She was diagnosed as having AIDS several months later after developing unusual symptoms. The distraught father submitted to testing and was found to be HIV positive. He then admitted to being actively bisexual.

The extremely ill child was admitted to a large, renowned teaching hospital, and there received the finest and most intensive care that scientific medicine had to offer. Still, after six weeks of extensive therapy there was no improvement and the parents were advised there was nothing more that could be done for their daughter. In despair, they took her home to die. As her symptoms became unmanageable, they sought other help and found my friend.

This healing practitioner went to the patient's home where the terrified parents were attempting to cope with a screaming child, obviously in pain, who could not eat because of Kaposi's Sarcoma of her mouth (a cancer commonly affecting the skin and alimentary tract of AIDS patients). She tried walking the baby, attempting to calm her, but that did not help. Finally, reaching into her mind for anything that might help, she had the parents fill the bathtub with warm water, and got into the tub with the baby, petting and soothing her and offering her sips of warm milk. Eventually, the baby calmed down and went to sleep.

The parents finally had time to ask, "What, if anything, can be done?" The healer admitted she really did not know. She then told the parents she first needed to find out from the child if she wanted to live or had decided to exit. To this end, she sat quietly with the baby for awhile, meditating and trying to receive some message from the child's soul or spirit, until she was finally convinced that the child wanted to survive. She then agreed to do everything within her capability to help in the healing process.

This valiant healing practitioner returned daily for several months, spending hours each visit doing whatever was necessary to nourish and nurture the infant. She spend time daily in the family pool with the child, soothing and comforting her. She offered the child tiny amounts of several Chinese herbal medications which she thought might be helpful, allowing her to accept or reject them.

The child began to improve. Her temperament calmed, she gained weight and her Sarcoma lesions disappeared. One of the biggest problems was re-bonding her to her mother, but after approximately six months the child's health had been restored, and the family was able to continue the nurturing process on their own. At last report, this child was six years old and normal in every way.

Now I do not mean to be disparaging about the care available at a fine medical facility, but there are some things about which allopathic medical practitioners, such as myself, simply have no knowledge. Modern antibiotics and other scientific medical treatment proved to be ineffective in helping this child. I do not know what part Chinese herbal medicines and Eastern therapeutic touch techniques played in her recovery. Personally, I believe she was healed by Love, with the help of someone who was willing to give it unconditionally. So far, we do not have any scientific instruments to measure this powerful energy.

I believe we could reach agreement among those in the healing profession that there are some unknown ingredients within each person that have either a stimulating or depressing effect on the healing mechanism, the immune system. It is essential to connect with and empower these important internal healing forces. We cannot be content to simply insert tubes and needles and pump in nourishment and chemicals and use cold, non-feeling machines to give life support. Touching, caring, transmitting optimistic thoughts, healing mental images, and loving energy to the patient, are all powerful healing medicines; extremely valuable and cost effective, available to all and unlimited in supply.

Perhaps we can agree on a more inclusive and nonspecific definition of <u>HEALING</u> as "*a process originating within a patient which moves him toward a state of health, and which may be enhanced or hindered by numerous outer influences.*"

Definition Of Disease

When one plans treatment for a disease, this treatment is naturally based on one's definition of the disease. It seems logical that if this definition is limited, then the treatment options will also be limited. For several hundred years, disease has been viewed as an abnormal physical condition. Therefore, the search for the cause and cure of illness has naturally been focused on the physical realm. Perhaps we should expand the boundaries of our definition and thus of our treatment options, because there is abundant evidence that mental, emotional, and spiritual factors also have important, causative roles in the creation of illness and in our ability to maintain health. These non-physical factors may be important in helping one avoid, combat, or possibly even to release, illness. Even though these influences are not physical and cannot be accurately weighed, measured, or looked at under a microscope, it seems naive to brush them aside and ignore them as though they were nonexistent, unimportant, or without impact on us physically.

Indeed, for many illnesses, the causes may lie primarily in these non-material realms. Physical symptoms or deformities may only be the visible manifestations, while the real sickness or unhealed area lies hidden somewhere within the emotional or mental or spiritual portion of one's being. If this is true, then treating or correcting only the physical problem will give only superficial or temporary relief. It will then be just a matter of time until the underlying disease process manifests itself again with the same or possibly even more serious physical symptoms.

At first glance, broadening our understanding of disease to include the nonmaterial realms of the mind, emotions and Spirit may seem to be adding complexity to an already complicated problem. However, if one looks only at our research into the physical causes and cures of disease, one can see that this has led us on an increasingly complex journey. It seems that each new discovery opens up an ever larger panorama of unanswered questions. I am sure researchers love this, as there is an ever expanding list of areas needing investigation.

No one is denying that amazing and significant discoveries have certainly been made and our knowledge of physical disease and treatment options has increased tremendously. But there has also been a quantum increase in the recognized scope of what we do not know. Each discovery seems to open a wider door into the unknown realm of limitless possibilities, with no bottom in sight. Perhaps by broadening the scope of our research to include non-physical causes and treatments, we will find some common denominators of illness that can focus and simplify our understanding and treatment of disease, rather than making it ever more complex.

Perhaps our investigation of disease has been focused on the wrong place – at the effect level rather than the causal level. We have been looking at the leaves and flowers and fruit of the disease tree, and we need to examine its trunk and roots and perhaps even more profoundly, its seed. We have been so fascinated by the appearance of disease at the effect level that an inordinate amount of our investigative resources and energy have been concentrated here. We have looked at everything outside ourselves – microbes, toxins, the environment. We have not adequately searched inside our minds, where we just might find the seeds of our discontent and eventual destruction. Could it be possible that the root cause of disease is to be found in the mind? It is obvious that external factors play key roles in illnesses, but maybe physical illness is not manifested unless the "soil" of the mind is in a state of dis-ease.

Looking into the mind for the errors of perception that may lead to disease is nothing new, but it has had a limited acceptance among the scientific community. I think it is time for us to openly include this non-physical realm in our area of exploration as we search for the perpetrator of disease.

In an attempt to promote agreement between all interested parties, I would like to suggest the following definition of <u>DISEASE</u>: *"any variation from the completely harmonious functioning of an individual on all levels of his being including body, mind, and spirit."* Perhaps this broader, non-confining definition can stimulate a more open-minded search for the elusive perpetrator of disease.

CHAPTER 6

AM I MORE THAN THIS PHYSICAL BODY?

If we are going to change our concepts about health, healing and disease to include not only the physical body, but also the mind and the spirit, then most of us are going to have to work on changing our belief about our own identity. In order to accept that there are advantages to looking for health anywhere other than in the physical realm, one must truly believe that there are such other realms. One must also believe that this "I" that I am interested in keeping healthy is something more than simply this physical body. Literally, we need to ask of ourselves, "Who am I?", and then do our best to find an answer.

The Harmfulness Of Body Identification

THE EFFECT ON THE INDIVIDUAL

Most of us identify ourselves as only physical beings. So how is this affecting us? Why would one wish to change this way of identifying himself or herself?

If I believe that I am only a physical body, then I have every reason to feel isolated and afraid. If I identify myself as a body, then I am subject to being harmed by the myriad natural forces and circumstances constantly surrounding me, over which I have little or no control. I am doomed to a life of insecurity, scarcity, pain and suffering, sickness, and eventual death. With this belief, it seems inevitable to me that I must live in fear and be constantly on the defensive. All the policemen and doctors and bank vaults in the world can't give me security.

We all recognize this distressing, defensive way of going through life. In fact, this is the level on which we operate most of the time. We have even given a name to this unpleasant existence, calling life a "rat-race." We sometimes try to hide or to run away. We take vacations to get away from it all, and we tell ourselves to "stop and smell the roses," but it seems impossible to escape completely from this insane, hectic, fearful drama. Even when we are at the seashore or in the mountains, there is an ominous, subconscious uneasiness. (Did I leave the stove on? I wonder what is happening to the stock market? Are the kids OK? Do you think this plane is safe?) Somewhere within there is a continuous sense of impending danger, always keeping the system poised and armed to do battle with all the forces that surround us and our loved ones, which threaten to crush or disrupt our vulnerable lives. What a strain! It is no wonder that we get ulcers, have nervous breakdowns, and feel "sick and tired' so much of the time.

As the process of editing and rewriting this manuscript was occupying my mind yesterday, I received a telephone call to inform me that the son of some dear friends had been killed in an automobile accident. This young man was their eldest child, and had graduated only two months ago from West Point

Military Academy. Now he is dead. All the hopes and expectations for his life have been dashed to the ground and
extinguished.

When I hear news like this, it is almost like a wave of nau-
sea passing over me, as I emotionally relive the experience of
our own daughter's death. I also again feel the despair that
wrenched my guts a few years ago when I learned that the son
of a lifelong friend and cousin had taken his own life by blowing his brains out with a shotgun. I feel the pain of watching
helplessly as the physical life of my sick father ebbs away. Even
though he is ninety-seven, I still do not want to let him go.

Reading the newspaper this morning about all the different
ethnic groups, religious groups and nationalities fighting and
killing each other, and the natural disasters, accidents, murders
and other atrocities, is very depressing. I have a tendency to
throw up my hands and shout into the void..."Where are You,
God? Don't You care?"

Viewed from our limited perspective, these tragedies do not
make any sense at all. Life, if seen as only life in this body and
on this earth, appears to be total insanity. We do not have eyes
in the back of our heads, and we cannot predict the future. It is
literally impossible for our bodies to be safe all the time.
Therefore, if we allow ourselves to think too much about the
potential dangers facing us, we will likely soon go crazy with
worry. Some people do this, and are diagnosed as paranoid and
finally lose their ability to function productively.

Since one cannot possibly function effectively while being
worried all the time, our common defense is to do something to
distract our minds. Most of us do this by keeping ourselves busy,
using every imaginable task or diversion. We find it intolerable
to have nothing to do, even for a short period of time. This

philosophy of staying busy has become a human addiction. Our belief in being only a physical body, with the unavoidable stress that accompanies that concept, has literally made us into compulsive human *doings* rather than human *beings*.

THE EFFECT ON SOCIETY

As a society of vulnerable bodies, we have recognized that individually we are unable to defend ourselves at all times against all the known and unknown threats to our existence. Therefore, we have surrounded ourselves with all sorts of protective inventions and institutions, and given our power away to them. To all these protective mechanisms that we have created, we have said, "We admit we are unable to care for ourselves. We now give you the responsibility for our well-being." These include governments, armies, police, judicial systems, churches, schools, etc. Most pertinent to this discussion, it includes our health care system.

THE EFFECT ON HEALTH CARE

Our society has made the decision that individually we are powerless against the forces of sickness. We have agreed to turn over the responsibility for our health to someone else, namely the medical establishment. Under this umbrella label I include all those who are willing to accept this job, including modern scientific medicine and all the alternative fields. There are plenty of volunteers, because we are willing to pay very dearly for this service.

I speak from my experience as a member of the scientific medical community. They have taken this responsibility for the welfare of our bodies quite seriously. They have dedicated themselves to service, organized their efforts, and undertaken massive amounts of research. They have made great strides in combating various forms of illness, and have even eliminated some. But perhaps the successes of the modern Western scientific medical establishment have been a bit intoxicating. There has developed a rather egotistical view that the scientific medical establishment invented and owns the healing process. The general public has largely accepted this view, and has lost sight of the fact that it is actually themselves doing the healing.

Having given our power away to those who would protect us, and having paid dearly for this protection, we are quite happy as long as things are going well and we are furnished wonderful "magic bullets," like antibiotics or kidney transplants or chemotherapy, (or cranio-sacral adjustments, acupuncture, herbs, or other 'alternative' treatments) that keep us feeling safe. On the other hand, it is not surprising that we feel betrayed and powerless when our hired protectors finally run out of ways to save us. This happens often when the doctor, who has been elevated in our minds to the position of a Shaman, finally makes the dread pronouncement that there is no hope, that no more can be done.

Some people accept this disturbing news quietly and simply give up, much like receiving a curse from a voodoo witch doctor. I have seen patients who literally die of the diagnosis. They have been living quite productive lives in spite of having a slowly growing cancer for years, and suddenly they have a diagnosis and it is like a death sentence. They quit doing the things that they enjoy, retreat from life, make a will, and die.

Others refuse to accept a hopeless prognosis and they seek other opinions and alternative solutions. Some do what this book is recommending and look for the deeper meaning of their illness, change their minds and their lives, and truly live until they die, now or later.

Still others react by becoming resentful and antagonistic. These angry patients feel abandoned and disenchanted, and they vent their frustration and hostility in the form of criticism, sarcasm, and even lawsuits against the medical establishment. It is ironic that the very ones who have been trying to play the role of rescuer are now identified by the victim as the cause of their problem!

As the end approaches, the ailing person who has identified strongly with his/her body frequently become frantic in the search to find something else "out there" that can be his/her salvation. These unfortunate 'victims' easily fall prey to charlatans who pose as healers, but whose only interest is in emptying their pocketbooks. The dreaded ending, the fear of which is causing so much panic, is the death of who and what one believes he is, namely a physical body.

Identifying too strongly with the physical body leads to all sorts of excesses in the medical care system. Are we not seeing at the present an exorbitant misuse of our medical resources on expensive life-sustaining technology that does not contribute to the quality of life, but is based solely on the fear of physical death?

Patients and their families, and their physicians as well, rarely have the courage to say, "Stop, this is enough!" and then to stand back and accept the inevitable. Why is this so hard to do? Because we still see ourselves as finite physical beings, with a limited life and no future beyond our physical bodies.

This focus on the physical body has even been carried into the realm of the ridiculous by some few with unlimited funds who go so far as to have deceased bodies frozen, in the hope that some day technology may find a way to restore life!

The medical system is currently being severely criticized and scrutinized because of its escalating cost. Many think that changing the system will be the answer. All the changes that I read about or hear discussed amount to nothing more than changing the outer form of the system, and in my opinion, this will not have any lasting benefit. Whether the system is free enterprise, socialized medicine or business-run medicine through HMOs, there will be no significant change as long as our focus of treatment is to save and protect the physical body.

For hundreds, maybe thousands of years, we have locked ourselves into a belief system that is based on a core concept which is erroneous. I believe a basic change must occur at this inner core. In order to have a more effective health care system that is caring but does not leave us powerless, we must change our basic concept. We are not simply physical bodies. Each of us has an identity that goes beyond the physical and extends into eternity.

To summarize, I have discussed the idea that the basic flaw in our search for health and security is that we see ourselves only as physical bodies. The medical care system also identifies us this way, and their diagnoses and treatment are focused accordingly. Out of fear and our perceived need for protection we have given our power away to persons and things outside ourselves that we think will keep us safe. This hasn't worked, because our bodies and everything else in the phenomenal world are constantly changing. If we see ourselves as only phys-ical beings, and safety is equated with permanence and lack of change, then we can never really be safe. As spiritual beings, on the other hand, we are part of an unchanging reality and our safety can never be threatened.

To make some sense of all this, the questions we need to answer now are: "How can we learn to see ourselves differently?" and "How can we take our power back?"

Finding
The Solution

CHAPTER 7

CHANGING
OUR IDENTITY

There is a statement in *A Course in Miracles* which reads "I am not a body. I am free, for I am still as God created me.[1]" I remember how startling this statement was to me when I first read it. I had always identified so closely with this physical self. The more I thought about this new idea, however, the more intriguing it became.

What a difference it would make if we knew that our being-ness was something far greater than a vulnerable human body! If we could become convinced at the deepest foundation of our belief system that we are more than physical bodies; if we could become secure in the knowledge that our true being, the essence of who we are, is something that is not physical, and not subject to change or the threat of destruction; if we could know that we are safe from any real harm, then we should have nothing to be anxious or fearful about and we would be able to live our lives in peace and harmony. Surely this spiritual concept would have a profound effect on our mental, emotional, and physical health. Let us examine this idea more thoroughly.

Letting Go Of Fear

I believe that each of us, whether we admit it or not, harbors a deep fear of dying, of giving up this physical existence and launching into the unknown...perhaps of being annihilated, of ceasing to exist. Letting go of that fear is not so easy for me, and that seems to be true for many others as well.

I have observed during my treatment of many terminally ill patients that most are terrified at the idea of leaving their bodies. It does not seem to matter how much physical suffering is taking place or how disabled they have become. Physicians and nurses know how difficult it is to treat a person who is terrified, and how poorly one responds to any treatment when fear and panic have taken over.

On the other hand, those who face the possibility of death with calmness or equanimity are not only easier to treat, but also respond more favorably. These fortunate (or perhaps enlightened) patients relax, and either get better or gently pass on. It has been my observation that in most cases where this inner peace exists, it is based on a strong conviction of one's non-physical, eternal nature.

People with life-challenging illnesses are wonderful teachers. I facilitated a support group for persons experiencing critical diseases for two years at the Loren Quinn Institute, and continue to do so at Getting Well, Inc. I am still amazed to see the healing that occurs as these participants work through their fears, especially those dealing with their mortality. It seems that becoming able to let go of fear and attaining a state of healing inner peacefulness can be learned but not taught, and depends upon each person individually making this effort for him or her self. The process, which I have observed repeatedly, is based on letting go of old restrictive concepts, including the fearful idea that one is merely a physical body. This letting go frees the mind to re-identify with the true essence of one's being, which is immortal. I believe that Ted's experience is an excellent example of how this can be accomplished.

Ted's Story

Ted was in his early 40s when we first met. He and his wife, Julie, had been married about ten years, following a short, romantic courtship in which each had immediately recognized the other as life-mate. Ted was an architect and a gifted artist. He was also a very introverted loner who preferred isolating himself in his own world of architectural and artistic creations.

Julie, on the other hand, is a highly extroverted person. This difference in personality types resulted in some frustration in the marriage, and over the years the couple had grown apart, interacting less and less. Ted consumed large quantities of beer daily, smoked heavily, and used marijuana liberally. He was a reluctant partner in any outgoing venture. Julie maintained her family connections, and remained involved with her many friends and social activities. Julie was Jewish in upbringing and tradition. Ted had completely divorced himself from any religion, he was agnostic and disinterested in spiritual concepts.

There were no warning signs of illness except for a mild cough. One day Ted coughed up blood, and at Julie's urging he had a chest X-ray, which led to other studies. After a full day of various X-rays and CT scans, Ted was given a radiological diagnosis of "inoperable lung cancer." This diagnosis was confirmed by bronchoscopy and biopsy during the next few days. Ted was advised to have radiation therapy and chemotherapy, but was told that these were only palliative and that his prognosis was very poor, with a life expectancy of only about six months.

Summoning resources from deep within himself, Ted chose not to quietly fold his tent, but instead to fight for his life, and Julie fully supported him in this decision. They committed all their time, energy, and finances to the quest for his recovery. He underwent the recommended treatment, and, in addition, read everything he could find about cancer in general and lung cancer in particular. He immediately stopped drinking and smoking either tobacco or marijuana. He sought the advice of other physicians, nutritionists, and alternative or complimentary therapists.

Ted and Julie also investigated various religions in their search for healing. They became more open to different forms of prayer, meditation and other spiritual practices.

Also at about the same time, shortly after starting his medical treatment, Ted and Julie began attending an Attitudinal Healing support group at the Loren Quinn Institute which I facilitated on a regular weekly basis. They participated enthusiastically and openly, and their journey was an education for us all.

Whenever there was a problem, they approached it with determination, optimism, and imagination. For example, when the chemotherapy made him extremely nauseated and none of his prescribed medication helped, Ted visited a Chinese herbal specialist whose unorthodox remedy was immediately effective.

We were privileged to watch as both adjusted to living again, following this traumatic change in their lives. It took Julie a few weeks to stop crying, and a while longer for Ted to open his tightly closed personality. We saw their relationship heal as they extended themselves for each other. Ted became outgoing and much more able to show his lovable nature. He reached out and repaired the damage to many friendships that had been abandoned over the years.

Ted began seeing a hypnotherapist who was helping him learn visualization techniques, and together they dealt with some of his difficult childhood issues. Once, he surprised his hypnotherapist by requesting that he would like her to help him see and feel the healing power of God. The therapist cooperated by helping Ted direct his attention deep inside himself. Here he suddenly discovered a light so bright and powerful that it was almost overwhelming. The vision was accompanied by an intense feeling of peacefulness, love, and a sense of oneness encompassing everything. As is so often the case with those who have transforming experiences, it was difficult for him to describe, but from that day on he never doubted the existence of God, and commented often that there was no way that any disease could withstand such a powerful loving Force.

Another day Ted reported to us an experience of a "visitation" by his long-deceased father. Ted had carried in his memory many incidents with his father during his childhood which he felt were abusive or at least unjustifiably harsh, and he harbored a great amount of unresolved anger and confusion regarding their relationship. He recounted to the group his meditative experience of "traveling" with his father in a lucid, dream-like state to re-visit all the incidents of his childhood. Together, he and his father watched these scenes being played out again. This time, instead of being a child-participant in the drama, he observed, as an adult with his father by his side. His father explained to Ted how he had seen each of the situations, and Ted was able to see the love that was behind his actions, which he had been unable to see as a hurting child. This resulted in a complete healing of their relationship. Remarkably, this healing occurred years after his father had died. Terry told us that his father visited him frequently after that, and they had long, comforting talks together. Fantasy? Vivid imagination? I believe it was real, whatever that is. What was real was the result—a very profound emotional and spiritual healing and a lightening of Ted's enormous burden.

Ted lived for over two years after his diagnosis. He had a seizure and was found to have brain metastases. He underwent more X-ray therapy and his symptoms regressed for a while, but his condition gradually deteriorated. Near the end he had difficulty communicating. He became partially paralyzed on one side and required a wheelchair, but for as long as possible he continued to attend our support group. Later, we visited him at home, then at a Hospice house. He never lost his ability to reason, his light-hearted sense of humor, or his peace of mind. Just before his death, he instructed Julie to have a party instead of a funeral and to play calypso-reggae music, which he loved. He warned her, with a gleeful sparkle in his eyes, that if she did not follow these instructions, he would not come! She did as he wished, and the gathering was a joyful and healing experience for everyone. I'm certain Ted was there enjoying himself and the many friends and family who came to love him.

Ted's case demonstrates the striking result of identifying with the spiritual part of one's being, and how this affects true healing. Once he accepted his true, eternal identity, he became more of an interested observer of the things that were happening to his body rather than being anxious and alarmed. Sure, there were times when he forgot and he would become depressed and sad, and this was when he needed Julie at his side to reassure him. Julie also frequently needed his loving support.

No, his tumor did not disappear, and his body eventually died, but not before he had healed, or come to peace with, every facet of his life. Who can hope for more? Ted told us near the end that it did not matter to him whether he lived another day, a month or for years. He said he was finally content. He also said that he felt that the two years since he had discovered that he had cancer had been the only time since his early childhood that he had truly experienced the fullness of life.

Ted's disease woke him from a deep slumber. It awakened him to a totally new concept of his own identity. Because of the cancer, he searched for new answers and a greater reality and meaning of life, and eventually found them inside himself.

Certainly this concept of a spiritual identity that transcends the physical is not new; it is the message of the Resurrection of Jesus Christ. His physical body died, but Christ continued to live. The philosophy of all the world's leading religions stress the impermanent nature of the body and the eternal nature of the soul or spirit.

Our problem lies not in finding teachings to support this view, but in accepting this non-body identity as the solid rock on which we base our beliefs. Only there will it have any influence on the way we live our lives; only there can it effect our health in a positive way. Fortunately for us, many teachers who are leading extraordinarily healthy lives have discovered that we do not need to wait until we contract a terminal disease before beginning the search for our true identity.

I have wrestled with my own reluctance to truly believe as questions continuously arise. It surely seems that when one of our loved ones dies, they are gone. As I struggled with these thoughts the following story came to me and it helped my understanding and acceptance of the transitory nature of this physical existence, and encouraged my belief in the permanence and limitless freedom at another level of existence.

DAVE THE WAVE
By Jasper B. Becker, Jr., M.D.

It was a Sunday morning in September. The wind was blowing briskly and there were squalls in the distance. The tide was nearly to the sea-wall and most of the beach, where cars usually drive, was under water. The air was warm and the water temperature just right for wading. A few adventuresome surfers were out beyond the breakers, and I watched as they experienced some spectacular rides.

I waded out until the water was just above my knees. The force of the breaking waves was fierce and the undertow was very strong. I decided not to wade any deeper, but simply to relax and enjoy all the wonderful sensations.

As my mind became quiet, a story emerged about a particular wave, whose name was Dave. As I watched the breakers crashing to the shore, Dave told me his life story.

Dave was born in a thunderstorm just off the west coast of Africa, a product of physical and cosmic forces at first appearing chaotic, then gradually developing rhythm in an intimate dance, building slowly in intensity until Dave emerged as an identifiable entity, defining a long arc with endless depth beneath him, allowing comfort and running room, as he gained momentum and became aware.

At first, he was almost unnoticeable, several times nearly disappearing back into the sea. "I am" was his first conscious knowledge of existence. Over time, he grew aware of his shape, form, dimension, and of his will. His fight for life was not easy. As water moving through water, he was subject to every cross current. Every storm that formed above circled winds that beat at his now towering or sometimes barely perceptible brow. His will was strong, and he knew he must press on, determined to experience everything there was to being a wave.

"There are others," he knew next. Waves of all sizes, forms and amplitudes. Endless columns and cross columns chasing over and through the ocean.

Many shared the pride and growing strength he carried, and attempted to grow in prominence. Others didn't seem to take being a wave too seriously and made little effort. Dave learned judgement, and discounted them as weak, half-formed, pitiable entities. Often he was shocked to see these same waves, many miles and many days later, resurging with a force that he had not predicted. He learned.

Play was next. For days during these good times, he and his friends rolled, danced and cascaded across the sea, sometimes with their heads rising 15, even 20 feet out of the water.

At other times, as fierce storms with swirling winds threatened his prideful body, and vicious cross currents undermined his foundations, he knew fear, and it took a mighty effort just to hold himself together. And he grew.

Being a successful wave took a lot of effort. Dave became proud of his success and enjoyed pushing up his chest. Every now and then when he got higher than any of his fellow waves, he would tip his white cap, as he secretly hoped the others were a little jealous.

Dave wanted to be seen as the best wave he could be, but sometimes, when the journey became a little boring, he had to keep reminding himself that he was happy, and that how he looked and performed was really important.

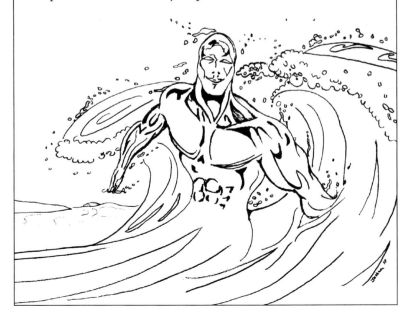

As he grew older, he grew in awareness. He began reflecting on his journey, contemplating his origins in the dark fathoms of ocean beneath him. There was a knot of fear here. That abyss could hold things, others, Non-waves! Other questions began to disturb him. Who was he, really, and where was he going?

His companions and he began to weave their own stories and sing their own deep songs, at first to soothe the dark thoughts and then to celebrate their victory over the darkness. And still he grew. He convinced himself that he was content and whole and strong.

It was morning, before dawn, when he heard the bizarre crashing sounds for the first time. Roaring crashes and the terrifying cries of his kind. And then the unthinkable. The resilient, bottomless sea of life beneath him, which he had always taken for granted, was disappearing. He began to feel his feet dragging, pushing, sliding over a shifting but much denser surface. He sang. He threw himself into his now familiar posture of defiant courage. Still the ocean floor tore at his foundations. With an ultimate exertion of his will, he towered higher, foam spilling over the peaked crest of his head. He sang louder, pushing with a desperate sense of urgency to even greater heights, until fear that had quietly haunted him since his birth, became one focused certainty.

Ahead, less that 50 yards away, was the final picture of his fear! After thousands of miles, hundreds of days, and the reassuring affirmations of countless of his kind, he knew that he was approaching the end of his long journey. He screamed. He roared with the force of a rogue elephant and the sound of ripping mountains "NOOOOO! DON'T LET IT END! I want more! I'm not finished yet! Is this all there is?"

As he crashed into the gently sloping white beach, he felt his whole being disappearing. His thrusting broad base eroded on the smooth rock and worn coral as his curling white crown sizzled out onto the flat sand. He felt he was losing his identity, and being annihilated forever! How he hated it as he became smaller and weaker. He finally was forced to surrender as he washed onto the beach exhausted.

For a moment he was overcome with darkness; but, to his surprise, it passed. He still "was," but where? How? No sense of struggle, no driving onward now. Indeed, nothing to drive with–no

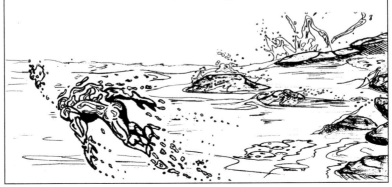

feet, no body, no crest. He rested there, but slowly he began to appreciate an enlarging sense of wholeness as the undertow pulled him into deeper waters. His consciousness seemed to expand as he slowly mingled with sea. He found the sensation quite pleasant, so he began to relax and just let himself go with the flow. "I am," he knew again, with surprise, even though he was unable to define his once familiar limits.

He looked upward and could see the turmoil on the surface. He had compassion for the frightened, helpless feelings of the other waves, who were crashing overhead. He tried to reassure them and share his newfound sense of peace. He shouted out to them "Look! Look at me! I've been through it and I'm still OK!", but they were so intent on the swirling world around them that they could not hear him. He ceased his calling as each joined him in turn.

Dave became more and more peaceful as he flowed deeper and deeper back into the sea. He was amazed to discover that though he had lost his identity as a wave, this is no longer important to him. He now became conscious of being something much greater. Instead of only the surface, he now had the whole of the ocean to explore. His terrifying fantasies about the ocean were dispelled, as he began experiencing a boundless sea of indescribable variety and beauty. He was ocean, wave, current, all and none of these. He was home.

As Dave reviewed his life from his new perspective, he realized that he had merely thought he was a wave. He saw now that all he would have had to do at any time was to look more deeply, and he could have seen that he was really a part of the sea all along. He remembered how hard he had struggled at being a wave, a big wave, because it had seemed so important at the time. He had kept himself busy posing and posturing, so as to look good to the others, who also thought they were waves. He relaxed in the glorious wonder of the great relief of existing in the flow–rather than in the struggle of trying to create his form as a separate wave. He was happy.

The End

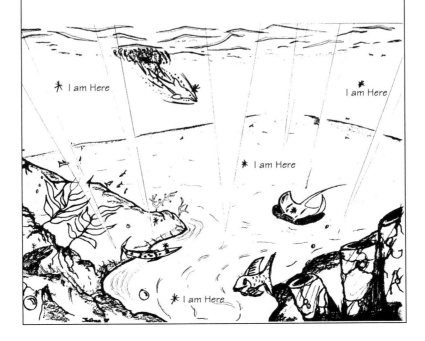

An Awakened Awareness

We have been addressing the issue of changing our concept of our identity from that of a physical body, with all its frailties and limitations, to the a vastly larger concept of a spiritual identity which is unlimited, indestructible, and eternal. Many reach this state of inner knowing through the teachings of religious institutions. For others, it may come through intellectual reasoning. Others acquire it through illuminating transformational experiences, intuitive mental imagery or personal communication with a Higher Source. Some may not discover this Greater Self without undergoing some life-changing tragedy. Others may never be open to question or experience anything like this during this physical life, but I believe they too will have this absolutely splendid revelation in a different time and place when they are ready. I think it is important, however, to make this discovery now, while we are on this physical plane and struggling with this 'here and now' existence. Doing so makes this journey so much more pleasurable.

An awakened awareness of this greater Identity also answers the second question, which I had posed as critical to our health: "How can we get our power back?" Every day I see examples of persons who have reclaimed their internal power. One can find these people anywhere, but they may not be noticeable unless one looks in areas where severe physical and emotional testing is occurring. My experience has been mainly in hospitals, and in support groups for those grieving personal losses, undergoing traumatic life experiences, or dealing with life challenging illnesses. You can recognize those who have reached this plateau of confidence in their higher Identity, because they sail through the troubled waters of life fearlessly.

The ones I know who have attained this splendid level of knowing are caring and giving, and seek to join with others. They are not afraid to participate fully in life. They find enjoyment, experience pleasure and also pain, and are also subject to emotional upset and bodily physical change and deterioration. They do not deny their humanity, but accept its limitations. When ill, they seek medical assistance and cooperate with scientific and alternative healers, but do so only if their personal intuition feels "right." They don't resist being cared for, but find no need to give their power away by being dependent on other people, things, or establishments to make them feel safe and whole.

No one I know personally has perfected the art of always remaining in an elevated state of peacefulness. Everyone seems to get knocked back to earth on occasion. Even the "enlightened ones" may need the support of others at such times to regain their stability. However, those whose conviction is deeply rooted usually do not take very long to learn from their experience. They discover that some form of fear is blocking the perception of their inner truth. Once they work through the fear and rediscover that the true Source of their power is unchanged, the fear disappears and they return to a state of healthy inner harmony.

Chapter 8

What Is
The Mind?

In the previous chapter we have been talking about changing our minds about our identity. When we speak about the mind it is necessary to be as clear as possible about a somewhat unclear subject. The *American Heritage Dictionary* lists 13 definitions of mind, perhaps indicating some disagreement. Definition #1 defines mind as, "The human consciousness that originates in the brain and is manifested in thought, perception, feelings, will, memory, or imagination." Definition #2 states that the mind is "The totality of conscious and subconscious processes of the brain and central nervous system that directs the mental and physical behavior of a sentient organism." Both of these obviously equate the mind with the physical brain. Definition #3 says that the mind is "The principle of intelligence; the spirit of consciousness regarded as an aspect of reality: mind over matter." This seems to indicate that mind is spiritual in origin. Down at #12 there is the concept of the Capitol 'M', Christian Science Mind: "The Deity, regarded as the perfect intelligence ruling over all of divine creation." Here, Mind, with a capitol M is referring to a higher consciousness. A *Course in Miracles* uses the term mind to represent "the activating agent of spirit, supplying its creative energy."[1]

Thus there seem to be two schools of thought: one asserting that the mind is a function or property of the physical brain and central nervous system, and the other seeing the mind as an intelligence outside of the physical brain, interacting with or being expressed through the physical brain in some unknown way.

Two Basic Functions Of The Brain

I try to simplify this a bit, bringing it down to something I can comprehend, and have come to my own conclusion that the brain basically serves two functions.

COMPUTER PROGRAMMING

One is these functions can be likened to a computer which processes and stores all the information coming to it through our senses and experiences. It is like a mega-mainframe, storing everything, including the memory of our emotional reactions to each experience. Some of this information is available to our conscious mind, but most is stored in our unconscious mind, carefully cross-indexed and matched up with interrelated data and emotions. Any new data coming in is instantly evaluated, categorized, and compared, using past stored information as the measuring stick for validity. Action messages are then sent to the rest of the body requesting a pre-programmed response.

To give an example: While driving an automobile, the light ahead turns red. Our foot is automatically taken off the accelerator and goes to the brake pedal, usually without these complex mental and physical processes coming into conscious awareness.

This computer-like activity of the brain allows us to function reasonably and rationally in this ever-changing environment, without having to be constantly bombarded by moment to moment demands for decisions. It's basic function is to preserve homeostasis: to maintain the status quo. This seems to be where we function most of the time.

Although this computer-like programming of our lives works most of the time, there is an uneasy awareness that we can never be completely effective in controlling everything, since we live in a physical world which is constantly changing. Therefore, we devote our time to the process of educating ourselves, trying to become expert in predicting, and thus being able to prevent, or at least be able to deal with, disastrous upheavals when they occur. We gather ever increasing quantities of information through our sensory experiences and our studies and store this into our computer-brain. In this way, we try to fine-tune our lives, programming in ever more appropriate responses, based on more and more experience or information. We scientifically analyze this data for its validity, trying to make our computer program as infallible as possible.

We have a problem, however, with using our brain in only this way. When we use only the stored information in our memory banks, we are continuously recycling only old information. We soon find ourselves stuck in circular behavior patterns that do not take into account the possibility of change or allow for growth. We are using information from the past to control the present, thereby effectively eliminating any hope for a better or different future.

When we encounter new problems or revolutionary ideas, we try to use old solutions where they won't work. We attempt to put the new material into belief structures where it doesn't fit. One solution often used by those with a "fixed" mind-set is simply to reject new information instead of reprogramming and constructing a new file. This is the chosen behavior of the extreme conservative, who dismisses all new information as worthless, and tries to live in the past.

TUNING IN TO THE MUSE

The second activity of the brain is to act as a transformer or conduit which allows expression of a higher mind, which is not an intrinsic part of the brain, but is outside the physical brain and is the source of new ideas or inspiration. This mind presents us with information from a higher, interconnected or Universal Source. This second function of our brains keeps us from getting stuck.

We might say that getting stuck, finding ourselves going around and around always ending at the same spot, is what happens when we are not "open minded." By that I mean when we are not using this second function of the mind and are blocking out the information available to us from a higher level.

Sometimes information from this higher mind comes like flashes of insight during periods of quiet contemplation. I have had it happen to me during crisis situations when I had run out of ideas and silently prayed for help. At other times unexpected solutions to problems seem to occur when one recognizes he is stuck, decides to "sleep on it," and awaken with new insight.

Albert Einstein humbly explained that his major discoveries did not come from his own analytical efforts but somehow simply appeared in his mind. Inspiration from this same higher source of intelligence may have been the mental connection that produced such immortal musical compositions as those of Bach, Beethoven and Mozart, and continues to influence creative contemporary composers such as Andrew Lloyd Weber. This source has been named the Muse, and surely the Muse was guiding some of the writings of such masters as Shakespeare or Thoreau, or the authors of our Constitution.

I would suggest that the only time we are really thinking is when we are using this second brain function to open our minds to a higher Source. The rest of the time we are mechanically running through the information stored in the computer part of our brain.

Everyone has the ability to connect into this greater wisdom. Unfortunately, we block this talent by staying tuned in to the noise of our computer-generated thoughts, or spending all our time attempting to gather information through reading, surfing the internet, watching TV, listening to Radio or audio tapes, attending seminars and just keeping our communication channels on-line and "busy." Practice of contemplative prayer or mindful meditation (going within the closet of the mind) uses "busy-ness" overcoming techniques, allowing us easier access to this inspirational source.

Is The Mind Separate From The Body?

The idea that the mind is separate from the brain and the body may at first seem rather preposterous to one who has not had occasion to give this much thought. It certainly did to me! However, we all seem to have some concept that this is true, for in our language we use expressions such as "going out of my head," or "my mind was wandering." Many, perhaps most, people have had personal experiences where their consciousness seemed temporarily detached from their bodies. These might have been lucid dreams, near death experiences (NDE's), out of body experiences (OBE's), vivid encounters with deceased loved ones, or simply day-dreaming.

More vivid documentation of the mind being separate from the body is available in accounts by persons who have had astounding experiences where they have been present in places distantly removed, or have seen and heard things that could have not been possible from the location of their bodies. For the more scientific minded, I would refer you to the works of Elizabeth Kubler-Ross, Raymond Moody, Brian Weiss, Gerald Jampolsky, and Depak Chopra, to name only a few. All of these are MDs of considerable scientific reputation. I mention that they are physicians because I think it is important to realize that there are already many within the health care system who are deeply interested in a more holistic view of man that encompasses vastly more possibilities than the purely physical.

There is a large body of ongoing research in the field of mind and consciousness. Bill and Judy Guggenheim's recent book, *Hello From Heaven,* is an extraordinary research effort in which they personally interviewed over 2000 people who claimed to have had after death communications with loved ones.

The Institute of Noetic Sciences[2] was founded by Edgar Mitchell, a former moon-walking astronaut, for the specific purpose of encouraging studies investigating the vast unknown of mind and consciousness. Some of the observations and results of these studies are truly astounding. This is not science fiction, but concrete information that is leading us toward a totally different concept, not only of health and disease, but of reality itself. How we learn to understand and use this information will undoubtedly have a profound effect on our health, and perhaps on the survival of the human race and life on this planet.

Learning To Use Our Mind For Healing

After years of feeling overwhelmed by the complexity of disease and its possible causes and treatments, I am inspired by the thought that the mind may hold simpler keys to the mystery of healing. I have come to believe that the power of the mind is essentially unlimited, and that it is the determining factor in the choices that we make and thus how we experience life. Philosophers throughout the ages have suggested that we are what we think. I would contend as well, that we are *more than* we think we are. Perhaps it could be our negative and limiting thoughts about ourselves which are the basis for our perceived deficiencies, disabilities, and our states of dis-ease.

Acquiring the skill to discover our erroneous, disease pro-ducing mental images with their associated negative thought patterns, then rooting these out are realistic and extremely worthwhile goals. Achieving these goals will allow more har-monious interaction between the higher mind, the brain, and the body and result in a calming of our fearful emotions, increasing enjoyment of life, and improved healing and health in our physical bodies.

CHAPTER 9

HOW DID I BECOME
WHO I THINK I AM?

Where do these disease-producing images in our minds come from? Perhaps the following discussion of the development of our self-image will lead to a better understanding.

Dr. Jeckle and Mr. Hyde

Have you ever experienced a sudden shift from a relatively peaceful state of mind to that of an enraged beast, just because someone made a sarcastic comment or jumped in line ahead of you? Everyone has this tendency toward volatile shifts in emotions, though some to a greater degree than others. Most of us seem to be just one step from the jungle of our most outrageous emotions. We usually haven't a clue where this rage comes from, and when it happens, we can usually conveniently point a finger at someone or something else as the cause of our violent reaction. This gets us off the hook for awhile, but when the same pattern happens over and over in different circumstances, we finally have to face the reality that this reaction is coming from inside ourselves, and take responsibility for it. What is this hidden inner unpleasant part of ourselves? Where does it come from? Why do we not see it all the time?

The Cloak Of Innocence: The Big Cover-Up

Most of us spend our entire lives constructing and repairing and perfecting an identity which we like to see as our ideal selves, and which we prefer to present to the world. We want a presentable outer personality. We need a mask that shows to others and to ourselves, "I am OK." We are generally pretty successful at manufacturing this outer cloak of innocence. Deep down, however, most of us would admit that it is really a disguise, covering up a lot that is not so perfect.

This work on the outer facade may take many forms. Some of these might be: becoming a people pleaser, earning more degrees, pursuing financial success, leading charitable causes, being a church workaholic, spending hours each day sculpturing the perfect physical body, or being obsessed with excelling in sports–whatever it takes. I'm not saying these things are wrong, but one needs to be very clear with him or her self, and not be doing them for the wrong reason. The wrong reason is to reinforce the "cover-up" simply because one is fearful of looking deeper inside.

We fear losing the security this outer cloak of innocence gives us, so we try to make it as thick and impenetrable as possible. This external armor protects us from being quite so vulnerable, but it also limits our spontaneity, our creativity, and blocks our childlike uninhibited participation in life. In this way the heavy cloak we have built for our protection and security becomes our prison.

What We Want To Cover Up: Our Shadow Self

Beneath our cloak of innocence are all the false perceptions and erroneous opinions which we have accepted as the hidden truth about ourselves. This collage of mis-information was constructed from bits and pieces that we picked up here and there as the world convinced us we were ugly or inadequate or guilty or sinful. This hidden inner self concept is generally a miserable self-image. It is our dark side, our "shadow" side.

A lot of this false, negative information came from our erroneous interpretation of well-intended but poorly communicated comments by parents, siblings, peers, teachers, doctors or ministers trying to assist us in reaching for higher goals. Example: "You are so lazy you will never be successful." The intended message may have been "I love you and am concerned about you. I would like to see you trying harder," but it is what is heard by the receiver that is implanted in his brain: "I am a lazy good-for-nothing person."

Young developing minds must also be severely traumatized by simply experiencing life as a small defenseless child in a world of giants, and living in constant danger of being hurt by any number of terrifying machines, animals, illnesses, and other disasters. An environment which adults may accept as normal imprints innumerable frightening images of weakness and inadequacy within the mind of a developing young child. Also, the violence on our television and movie screens certainly cannot but accentuate the message that this is a fearful world, and I am told by psychologists that our brains store all this information as if it were real!

Little minds are unable to deal with all this frightful information being dumped into its developing consciousness, so in defense of itself, the mind pushes much of it into the subconscious. The subconscious mind dutifully files all this terrifying information away, and stores it as it was experienced: as the impressions of a frightened, defenseless child.

Burying this information is a great defense mechanism. It allows this struggling child to grow and develop in spite of what, if held continuously in the conscious mind, would be overwhelming. We still use this same defense mechanism as adults. When faced with too much threatening information, we often say to ourselves, like the classic line by Scarlet O'Hara in *Gone With the Wind*, "I'll think about that tomorrow." Unfortunately, we bury some unpleasant information or impressions so deeply that we do not ever deal with them, and they act like smoldering pockets of putrid infection that continuously release toxins into our lives.

Fear Of Exposure

It is the fear of exposure of these hidden impressions, the fear of allowing someone else to see these frightening, child-like beliefs we have buried within us, that blocks intimacy. For example, when a shy adult is trying to get his/her courage up to establish a meaningful relationship, this hidden negative inner child-like belief whispers defeating messages as: "He would not like me if he really knew me;" or, "Be careful what you say or she will find out how really stupid you are." Such negative self-talk may also limit us when we are considering applying for a job, or auditioning for a part in a play, or sabotage our efforts when attempting to lose weight or stop smoking.

The most hurtful negative impressions are those resulting from severe emotional, physical, or sexual abuse. These can cause the creation of an inner mountain of negativity and self hatred. This may account for some criminal behavior. This painfully negative self-opinion of such persons gives rise to thoughts like "Go ahead and pull the trigger. Everyone can already see you are bad and damned to Hell, and you can never change;" or, "You are so despicable that no one is ever going to love you, so if you are to satisfy your sexual cravings you may as well rape someone." Sounds horrible, doesn't it? Fortunately most of us are not so filled with self-hatred that we become murderers or rapists. We all have some negative opinions of ourselves, however. We develop these opinions quite early, and spend the rest of our lives trying to cover them up.

I hope the reader can visualize the picture I have tried to paint: An outer cloak of innocence, total control and tranquility, telling oneself and the world that "I am OK"; and an inner negative or shadow self which we have tried to bury into our subconscious that tells us "I'm not OK."

Emotional Hazards Of Maintaining A Facade

The painful emotions, which accompanied the unpleasant experiences we have stuffed into our subconscious cannot be so easily covered up. Although the buried memories may be out of sight, and seemingly out of mind, their emotional content is still very much alive. Even though we have plastered over the painful memories with our outer mask of innocence, there remain little sensory projections that protrude through the surface of our consciousness. These are like the triggering devices of buried land minds. Everyone has their own emotional tripwires, their own peculiar sensitivities, just waiting for the their own particular stressor to come along and blow their cover. I have heard or experienced so often, "I don't know what happened to me! I thought I had it all together, then he (she or it) showed up and I just fell apart!"

Some people are better than others at constructing an outer mask. Those who are not very successful at putting on a convincing front are usually considered failures in our society, which tends to reward outward appearances. These social "failures" leave inadequately covered areas in their outer masks and these are constantly eroding. These vulnerable people who are unable to effectively cover up their underlying feelings of guilt, shame, and inadequacy do not fit well into a society which is dominated by those who are more able to mask these very same feelings.

It may be comforting to know, if you are one of those persons who has never been able to construct a solid outer mask and frequently feels vulnerable, embarrassed, laughed at, shamed or ridiculed, that probably you are closer to the truth about yourself than those who have been more successful in building a convincing outer mask of competence and self-assurance.

Our culture, including many of our religious institutions, seems to encourage identification with the outer cloak of innocence, and to discourage any in-depth probing into the dark secrets underneath. We enjoy the illusion that we, and the person sitting next to us in the pew, working with us in business, or taking us out on a date, is the stable, sound, totally rational being that he or she seems to be. It always comes as a shock when a perfectly normal appearing person flies into a rage or otherwise acts out seemingly inappropriate behavior. Our natural reaction when this occurs is to immediately look for a way to excuse the incident and try to patch things up, so that in our minds this person can return to being the uncomplicated friend we think we know and whose behavior we would like to believe we can predict.

Attempts at covering up the eroded, vulnerable places in this outer mask may take the form of addictions. The use of addictive substances, or addictive behavior patterns (one may be a sex-aholic, golf-aholic, work-aholic, bridge-aholic, etc.,) are all forms of denial, allowing one to temporarily distract himself from the unpleasant images that are seeping out into conscious awareness. Unfortunately (or fortunately!) this addictive covering-up is only temporary, and requires repeated applications of increasing potency.

I have heard recovering addicts describe their problem as a "hole in the soul." A more accurate description of the underlying cause of addictions is that the addict is uncomfortably aware of a hole through the fabric of the outer mask, exposing his insecurities underneath. This hole is not really a hole or deficiency in the soul, but in fact is a potential opening into true awareness of the soul. Therefore, instead of covering over these openings, a more beneficial goal would be to acknowledge, accept, and explore them, as painful as this may seem.

Exploring these opportunities can be frightening and difficult, but sooner or later is has to be done because the only way to our truth is through our inner hidden fears. If we want to heal we must find the courage to go inside and expose these false negative perceptions of ourselves to the light of reason and truth. The alternative is to live a lifetime of denial, attempting outwardly to display confidence and competence while being filled with the uneasy awareness of buried insecurities and phobias which can erupt at any time. Maintaining the outer mask, or cloak of innocence, and refusing to go into and through the inner muck, severely limit ones ability to fully participate in life. This charade also extracts a heavy toll on our mental and physical health.

Searching For The Truth About Ourselves

If anyone reading this thinks that you do not have some buried doubts and fears, just think of the worst thing that could happen that would disrupt your tranquility. It may be losing all your money or your youthful beauty, going blind, developing cancer, or losing a child. More simply it may be baldness, being turned down when asking for a date, double faulting at set point, or coming in close contact with someone of a different color, nationality, religion or political party—whatever pushes your buttons. These buttons are examples of life experiences we try to avoid because they trigger those fearful anxieties and insecurities which we buried long ago, and wish would stay out of sight and out of mind.

Overcoming these self-imposed limitations to a full, healthy and happy life is a goal of many psychological therapies, including Inner Child work, Neuro-linguistic programming, Gestault therapy, Jungian analysis, Attitudinal Healing, Hypnotherapy, and others. A person who is struggling with unresolved painful emotional issues which have been repressed, can choose any of a number of techniques, but the main ingredient is a personal willingness to explore. No one else can do it for you. No therapy can resolve your personal issues if you are unwilling to look at them. One must walk through his/her own personal emotional minefield to be able to walk through life as a full participant without fear of intimacy.

Unfortunately, many go through life never seeing anything but false faces, their own and those of others, and unless some disconcerting incident occurs which forces one to look deeper, he or she never develops real intimacy. Being willing to look inside oneself, and perhaps even more frightening, opening oneself to someone else, is the true meaning of the word intimacy. This word could also be written, "into-me-see."

Beneath The Mask And The Muck... Finding Our True Selves

Recurring emotional distress, frustration and the inability to find permanent solutions may eventually lead one to stop pointing the finger of blame, to stop trying to fix something or someone out there, and to begin to look inside oneself where the real problem lies. As Carol Howe so beautifully points out in her seminars, the problem always lies within our own mind, and here is where correction is needed, and only here is it possible to find permanent solutions. She says that our perception of the outer world is simply a mirror-like reflection of what is going on inside us. Carol uses as an example a person who looks in a mirror and doesn't like what she sees. She realizes that it would be foolish to try to correct the problem by applying makeup to the mirror! It seems much harder to apply that same logic to our emotional problems.

Even when we do finally decide to look inside ourselves we are sometimes unable to see our way clearly to discover what corrections are needed. At those times, Psychological counselors can help us explore, understand, and come to peace with our inner hidden self-deceptions.

Transpersonal Discovery: Who Am I?

Transpersonal Psychology takes the process to the next, and most important level. The goal of this healing art is helping us discover the truly marvelous and lovable beings that we are, behind or beyond our artificial personality veils.

Gradually, as we learn to not be afraid of the imaginary bogey-men that we have hidden away, we no longer feel so vulnerable, and we find we no longer need such an impenetrable outer shell. We can afford to become more trusting, open, and intimate.

Eventually, our search for wholeness can even allow us to be thankful for the situations or persons that trigger the emotional explosions that uncover our buried fears. When the inner shadow has been exposed to the light of truth and revealed as the nothingness that it is, the outer mask is no longer needed, and the God-created beauty of our true Self shines through, becoming present and active in us and visible to others.

This internal self-re-evaluation, getting rid of errors of perception about ourselves and re-discovering our true value, is where healing occurs. Removing these internal errors of perception in myself, and observing the same happening in others, are experiences that remind me of surgically removing a malignant tumor. These mental corrections are even more life-saving.

Recently in one of our Attitudinal Healing group sessions, one woman experienced an obvious correction of perception. Her major physical problem was chronic and crippling pain in her legs from diabetic neuropathy. When asked to identify her major fear, she responded tearfully that it was the thought of

becoming an invalid, of having unusable legs or perhaps requir-
ing amputation. Having said that, she became quiet for a few
moments as a light seemed to dawn in her mind. She then
remarked that the word, "invalid' actually has two meanings. It
could mean being infirm physically, but it also meant being "invalid," or of no value as a person. Her real fear, she said, was not
so much of losing her legs, but of being invalidated! She realized that she had been basing her identity and her measure of
self worth on the physical condition of her body. It was plain to
see that she was breaking through to a new level of understanding of herself as a more permanent, powerful, and valid
being.

When all of our misperceptions, have been exposed as the
nothingness they are, what we find is our true identity: the
innocent inner being that God created, who has not changed.
From the brief glimpses I have had of the true Self, (mine and
others), this Real Self is totally healthy, loving, innocent and
magnificent!

CHAPTER **10**

THE EFFECTS OF OUR BELIEFS ON OUR IMMUNE SYSTEM

Setting The Stage

We have laid the foundation for a basic restructuring of our belief system. We understand there is some inner work to be done toward ridding ourselves of the false coverings, or false perceptions of ourselves. We now are somewhat accepting of the idea we have physical bodies but that we are more than bodies. We have begun to change our sense of identity. We have at least a longing to feel the essence of our being is something indestructible, unchangeable, eternal, good and God-like.

How does this lead to healing? It is easy to see this new-found sense of a greater identity leads to emotional healing. We become less vulnerable and have no need to react emotionally to the slings and arrows of life that had kept us in turmoil in the past. We feel powerful and whole because we know who we are! There is also a definite connection between what we think about ourselves and physical healing.

Some physical healings may be sudden and "miraculous," which by definition makes them unexplainable in scientific terms. I personally have no doubt these occur, and I think they are the result of a shift at some super-conscious level. I have no knowledge to understand or explain these healings which defy scientific logic. Perhaps when we finally, as a human race, come to identify with our Greater Reality, these healings will occur naturally and will no longer be a cause for wonderment. For the moment, however, I will concentrate on the healings we understand, and try to show how these are catalyzed by the perception of our True Selves.

Physical healing, even at its normal pace, seems miraculous. There are so many truly fascinating steps in this process that occurs naturally and effortlessly in our bodies. This type of healing is under the control of our immune system. Since it proceeds so silently it appears we have no ability to direct this healing process, but that is simply not so. Within recent years it has been shown without a doubt that there is a connection between the immune system and our beliefs, and the thoughts that arise from these beliefs.

Wow! This is a major insight, ranking right up there with the discovery that the world is round, or that germs cause diseases! How empowering it is to know that what we think can positively or negatively effect our body's health. It seems so "right" because we suspected it all along but no one would come right out and say it in scientific circles. Let us now examine this thing called the immune system more closely, and see how it is effected by our thoughts.

The Immune System

Our immune system is the guardian of our physical health. It is a very complex part of our physiology and is present throughout all of our body. The widespread nature of the immune system has contributed to the difficulty in forming a definitive concept about it, because it is not just one organ or set of organs. It includes the nervous system and its neuro-endocrine chemical message system, all bodily organs including the sensory organs, the blood and lymphatic system, the digestive system, reproductive system, musculoskeletal system, the skin, and even organs which were previously thought to be unimportant and disposable, such as the thymus, tonsils, spleen, and appendix. No organ, system, or even cell is excluded, for each has some function in the body's complicated self-defense mechanism, the immune system.

If there has been one benefit of the AIDS epidemic, it is its stimulation of the scientific study of the immune system. This system is extremely complex, involving all sorts of genetic codes, messenger chemicals, enzymes, targeting antibodies, killer cells, and a host of other factors being discovered daily. Comprehensive information filling many volumes is available in the scientific literature, and the surface has only been scratched.

Psychoneuroimmunology

The word "Psychoneuroimmunology" (PNI) has recently become commonly used. It is the study of the connection of the mind, the nervous system and the immune system. It is generally accepted that disease occurs due to an interaction of many causative factors. One essential ingredient for disease to manifest physically is an inadequate response by the body's immune system. Many detrimental events, such as exposure to various toxic substances, can cause the immune system to become weakened, but what is viewed as revolutionary by many is the notion that the immune system's response can also be affected by a person's thoughts.

There is no question in my mind that our thoughts have an effect on our bodies. I think most people accept that. I can simply think of squeezing a juicy lemon into my mouth and my salivary glands respond. I can worry about being late for an important appointment and my stomach pumps out hydrochloric acid. I can be angry and have hostile feelings toward someone and my adrenal glands respond by pumping out adrenaline and my blood pressure and heart rate go up. The thought-about person or situation does not have to be physically present, just the thought. On a more pleasant note, everyone knows how their own sexual organs respond to sensual thoughts, images or dreams.

In our everyday expressions, we state our belief in the relationship between our thoughts and our physical condition. How many times have you heard, or spoken yourself, statements such as: "My little brother (or child or mother-in-law) is a pain in the neck." "This new job just ties my stomach up in knots and is giving me ulcers." "My heart aches," or "My heart broke when she left." "I feel like I am carrying the weight of the world on my shoulders." "This anger is eating away at my insides." Our thoughts are being expressed as feelings within our bodies. It is not a great leap for most to accept that these thoughts are actually changing the condition of our bodies; that our bodies manifest what our consciousness holds. Similarly, our thoughts can enhance or depress the function of our immune system.

Thoughts And Emotions
Which Depress The Immune System

FEAR

What about fear thoughts? How do they effect us? For the answer just look at what we say about ourselves when we are afraid. "I was paralyzed with fear." "I was so frightened I froze in my tracks." "Fear completely immobilized me." "I am scared to death!"

When we have terrifying thoughts or experiences can there be any doubt but that our bodies get the message and respond? Kinesiology (the measurement of muscle strength associated with various thoughts) easily demonstrates that fearful or negative thoughts cause our muscle strength to weaken. It seems logical that the immune system responds to fear thoughts in the same way that the rest of our body does: by becoming weak, paralyzed, frozen, immobilized and shutting down in despair.

In 1933, this country was in the depths of a depression following the collapse of the banking system. One third of the country was unemployed. Bread lines were forming. There were riots and widespread political discontent and the seeds of a possible communist revolution were taking root. The clouds of war were again rising over Europe. Everyone was afraid. In his inaugural address to the American people, President Franklin D. Roosevelt said: "The only thing we have to fear is fear itself." He knew fear would hamper our ability to respond appropriately to the challenges ahead. His statement remains true for each of us today when we face our own private catastrophes. How we handle these fears determines our body's response to emotional and physical health challenges.

Fearful thoughts naturally arise when our sense of well-being is threatened. Our immune system's response depends on our beliefs...about disease, about life and death, about ourselves and who or what we think we are. Based on these and other beliefs, we have programmed our brain to orchestrate a bodily response. Are these programs vitalizing? Are they founded on a joyful will to live or are they self defeating, founded on despair? Will the response of our immune system be healing and overcoming, or will it surrender to disease?

Fear may block a person's recovery from illness and it can also make one more susceptible to the onset of illness. The effect of fear on the immune systems of animals and humans can now be measured scientifically thanks to medical technological advances. Experiments have been performed which exposed rats to a fearful, stressful environment from which they could not escape or protect themselves. These studies demonstrated that this stress caused malignant tumors to grow faster. There was also a measurable decrease in the production of the protective chemicals and cells of the immune system during fearful, stressful situations.

Some amount of stress is a normal and essential part of our lives, and stimulates us to move and take necessary action. For example, hunger, cold and loneliness are stresses that encourage us to search for food, clothing and companionship. But when stress is continuous and overwhelming, or when it is not appropriately handled, it can be destructive to our health by depleting our body's defensive resources and potentially opening the doorway for disease.

When disease occurs, the problem becomes compounded because the disease itself is stressful. This stress on top of stress is sometimes enough to do us in, so to speak. I have had patients who I believe literally died of the diagnosis of cancer, somewhat like the "straw that broke the camel's back."

When we are dealing with the stress brought on by the presence of disease, I think the usual reaction is fear. Let's try to identify a few of these fears other than the fear of dying. There is fear of pain and suffering. There is fear of not being in control of one's life, and related to that there is fear of being dependent upon someone else. There are certainly fears of economic disaster related to illness. There are any number of other fears. Some may seem ridiculous, but are nonetheless real to the one whose life is being crippled by them. One is the simple fear of being wrong, and this fear can influence a person to choose to be "right" rather than to be well. An example of this is the classic gravestone epitaph: "See, I told you I was sick."

Another person might have a fear of getting well because an illness furnishes something he or she thinks is needed. We can have a great deal of investment in our illnesses. One who has felt abandoned and neglected may only get the satisfaction of personal attention when he or she is sick, and may experience great emotional distress at the thought of no longer having this illness.

Another is the fear of loss of identity. One may have completely identified himself with the illness, and having let everything else go, would fear he would be "invisible" if he should give up the illness.

On a more materialistic level, and perhaps pointing up a defect in our social system with its overly zealous intent to throw money at all problems, the disability payment system may contribute to the prolongation of illness as the patient feels fearful of resuming a normal life and thus giving up a comfortable but crippling and enabling subsidy.

To make a point which I hope may offend only those who are deliberately abusing the system, I will repeat a recent joke that addresses this issue. It goes something like this: Three men were playing golf, and a fourth man joined them. He introduced himself as God. The other three scoffed in disbelief, assumed he was nuts, and challenged him to prove that he was God. One man had a damaged knee and walked with a limp, and "God" walked over and touched him and he was immediately healed. They were amazed. The second said he had long suffered from difficulty breathing and got short of breath on walking only a few steps. When he was touched by the newcomer, his symptoms immediately disappeared and he was able to run and do strenuous exercise without any difficulty. With that, the third man looked alarmed and stepped back, saying, "Keep away from me. I don't want you to touch me. I'm on disability!"

Our natural bodily healing mechanism is trying to keep us well and healthy, and it takes its directions from what we hold in mind. When our mind, for any conscious or subconscious reason, tells the body, "Don't get well!", the body and its immune system hear and obey.

When attempting to let go of fear, resistance naturally arises. It is quite common for a person to feel resentful and to say, "How can I possibly let go of these fears. They are not imaginary, they are real! I really am about to lose my house, and I really do have a cancer that is eating up my spine." There is no question that these types of fears are real. They are certainly real as long as one is only looking at what appear to be the facts from his singular perspective. The discouraged, fearful person is at the stage described in previous chapters where he is caught in a vortex of circular thought patterns: No matter how many times he mentally processes the information contained in his mind, he comes up with the same hopeless answer. He is stuck, and needs some help to find a way out. He needs a way to view his situation from a different perspective.

Mental health counseling and psychotherapy offered for patients with life-challenging conditions is focused on empowering the individual, by opening his mind to the possibility of new perspectives that can get him unstuck. The counselor does not have the answer for the patient, but helps guide the patient to his own best answer which lies hidden within himself.

This therapy sometimes involves story-telling. I would like to share a story about "going inside" to find answers in fearful situations.

THE CRAB TRAP
By Jasper B. Becker, Jr., M.D.

A crab trap is a cube shaped container, about three feet in height, made of chicken wire mesh. In its center there is a wire container for bait such as raw chicken or fish heads, food irresistible to crabs. There are four cone shaped openings, one per side, through the outer perimeter of the trap, like inverted funnels.

The outer end of each funnel is large and easy for a crab to swim into from the outside, and the bait can be seen through the funnel.

The small end is oval shaped and close to the bait near the center of the trap. This inner opening is just large enough to allow a crab to pass through.

Visualize Kathleen Crab, happy and carefree,

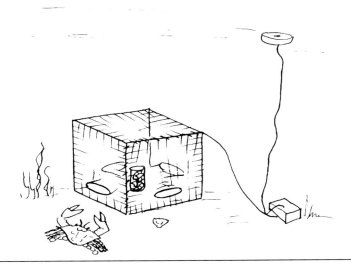

swimming along enjoying her freedom. She isn't extraordinary to the casual observer, but to those who know her she has a rather reserved personality. She isn't one to fight the other crabs for food, but has done OK just hanging back and taking the left-overs. Sometimes, she feels resentment toward the more aggressive crabs, but she holds this inside, as she is afraid of getting hurt if she asserts herself too much.

Suddenly, Kathleen catches a whiff of some delicious food nearby and becomes quite excited. She circles this big square wire container and sights the plentiful quantity of tasty looking food inside. It appears to be free for the taking, and without any forethought Kathleen swims right into the trap and begins to feed on the bait.

She eats until she is full, takes a little rest and then decides to move on. Much to her surprise she is unable to find her way out. In any direction that she swims, Kathleen bumps into the wall of wire.

Gradually she begins to comprehend that she is trapped. This does not seem so bad at first since the food is readily available, and the wire cage protects her from dangerous predators.

She spends her time between feedings searching for an escape route around the periphery of the trap. She spreads her long legs and claws out wide, trying to feel as much of the wall as possible. Her simple-minded concept is that if she is to find a way to the outside, it must obviously be through the outer wall of the trap. She cannot remember exactly how she got into the trap because her attention at that time had been so focused on the bait luring her inside.

As she looks outward through the wire mesh, Kathleen can see other crabs swimming by. She remembers longingly the beautiful freedom she is no longer able to experience. She comes to realize that eating is not the only important thing in life. She tries to get the attention of passing crabs in the hope they can help her find a way out, but they just drift by, uncaring, focused on their own needs and desires.

There are others crabs in the trap. Kathleen has become acquainted with some of her fellow prisoners. She has discovered she is not so alone after all. She had always thought she was so different, but now she is learning just how much they all have in common. Even though each one has a unique life story and different ideas as to just how he or she managed to get inside the trap, they have all ended up in the same place, and all are searching for a way out.

Occasionally, one of them mysteriously vanishes, and this encourages Kathleen in her belief that an escape route exists, heightening her interest in the search. Again and again, she inspects every single inch of the outer wall of the trap. Nothing! No openings are found anywhere.

After the food in the trap has run out, her search for an escape route becomes frantic. Her efforts are slowed as her muscles waste away and she feels her strength fading. Finally she can only cling to the trap wall, forlornly gazing at the beautiful world outside which is no longer hers to enjoy.

Suddenly, she sees a crab swimming by that she recognizes as having once been a prisoner inside the trap. She calls out desperately, and much to her relief this liberated crab hears her and swims over and asks if he can help.

"Oh, thank you. Thank you." says Kathleen. "Please tell me how to get out of this trap. I am starving for food and for my lost freedom. I know there must be a way out because I see that you are now on the other side of this wire and once you were inside with me. Please tell me where the secret doorway to my freedom can be found."

"Well," said the liberated crab, who was quite an intellectual, "it is like this," and he begins a long-winded discourse on the structure of the trap and the funnels and how the mechanics work, and what it all looks like from his present viewpoint, et cetera, et cetera. Poor starving Kathleen, who is about to lose her grip and collapse, exclaims in desperation, "Stop, stop. I am unable to understand! Please just give me simple directions so with my last bit of strength I may be able to escape"

"Of course," said the liberated crab. "Sorry I was running on so long. It is really quite simple. You

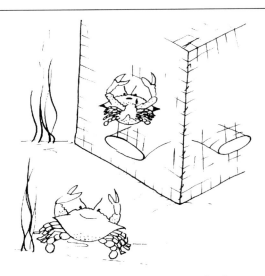

will not find the escape route through the outside wall of the trap, you must GO WITHIN..." And before he could explain further, a strong current whisked him away. Kathleen was left to ponder on the meaning of this strange instruction.

For a long time she was quite still. Many thoughts went through her mind. She became angry when she realized how hard she had struggled and how much valuable time she had wasted. She felt so hopeless because she had no idea what to do with her newfound instruction. Gradually, her grasping and clinging to the wire outer wall of the trap loosened. Finally, when she was no longer strong enough to hold on, she simply let go. She drifted around aimlessly for awhile, but finally she managed to extend one flipper, and she paddled ever so slowly until she came to rest near the center of the trap.

As though in suspended animation, Kathleen remained quite still there for a long time, too tired even to think. Her eyes were barely open, but gradually she began to notice that from this position something looked different. She opened her eyes wider, and she saw the openings that had escaped her attention all this time. Almost unbelieving, and afraid to get her hopes too high, she slowly paddled over to one of the openings. It was small, but she realized that if she oriented her body at just the right angle she could slip through. She folded her legs and her claws, and made herself as little as possible. With one tiny flipper she gently propelled her body through the narrow oval-shaped opening and outward, into the beautiful freedom of the open sea.

Kathleen recovered, but she was never the same again. She relished her freedom, and enjoyed every day. She stood up for herself when necessary. She had many other experiences, and grew to be old and wise. Whenever she faced a perplexing problem she would bury herself in the sand, fold up her legs, become quiet, and remember the instruction to "Go Within." As she would drift peacefully into the inner depths of her mind, she would eventually see again an opening that would lead her out of her dilemma.

The End

It is interesting that the derivation for the word cancer is from the Latin, *cancer*, which means crab.

Anger

Anger seems to be a separate emotion, but in truth it is only a reaction to fear. Eminent psychologist, author, and speaker, Dr. Wayne Dyer, uses a very descriptive metaphor to help us understand anger. He asks his audience the question, "What comes out when you squeeze an orange?" The answer, of course, is orange juice. Dr. Dyer then makes the point that just like the orange, when a person is squeezed, what comes out is what is already inside. We can understand better from this illustration what is happening to us when a situation or a person shows up in our lives and seems to make us boil over in a rage. The anger was already in there, and the thing or person that squeezed us did not cause it but merely was the activating agent that made it flow out.

All of us have special people in our lives that seem to push our anger button. If there is not an individual close to us who performs that function, we can readily find an ailment, politician, sports figure, racial group, ethnic group, or something else "out there" to blame for our frustration. This enables us to continue to see ourselves as an innocent victim, justified in our anger. Let me be clear in reiterating that it is not these people or things which are our problem. Our problem is inside us! The buried negative emotions that we already hold inside because we think ourselves unworthy, is what comes out when life "squeezes" us.

We do not understand why certain people or ideas affect us so negatively, but we feel the unpleasant emotional juice that comes out of us. Since the real source of this anger is buried in the subconscious where we are unable to see it, and are afraid to look, it is quite a natural response to project our anger and frustrations outward on others. Hitler very effectively used the

Jews as his scapegoat and probably never consciously realized that the thing he hated the most was himself.

We can fool ourselves for awhile with this technique, but the negative ideas never really leave their source, which is our own mind, and they continue to do their damage inside, sapping our strength and energy and diminishing our zest for life. They act like destructive laser beams with which we zap ourselves. This chronic bombardment by these harmful thoughts finally breaks down our immune system, and our bodies become more susceptible to illness.

Sometimes our emotional storehouse is so filled with the juices of anger, hatred, and resentment that it is impossible to be rational. Anger-releasing therapies, which depressurize this negative energy, are helpful. Alone, however, this releasing will offer one only temporary relief. Permanently successful therapy depends on following this anger release with precisely locating the source of this hateful emotional toxin. It can then be exposed to the light of reason, understanding and forgiveness. When this source is removed it makes room for the Elixir of Life that is naturally inside us, which is Love.

Grief

Anger is not the only emotion that fills us, and which we try to hide inside ourselves. Another is grief. How else can we explain the torrent of tears that sometimes is brought forth by a seemingly insignificant incident or word, or even a song or a scene in a movie? These events seem at times to be the triggers that burst the dam of restrained grief. Surely the human race has enough stored-up grief to cause another flood as severe as the great Biblical flood experienced by Noah. Forty days and forty nights would probably not be enough time for this rain of grief to pour out.

We may have simply pushed very grievous incidents aside and gone on about life thinking it was better to be strong, avoiding the natural process of grieving our loss. We could really befriend ourselves by finding a safe time and place, and then allowing ourselves the luxury of crying until there are no more tears. As this well of tears is released, one may be surprised at the discovery of the large number and variety of losses we never fully acknowledged.

Perhaps it is possible for our healing processes to literally drown in this unresolved grief, so if you are sick and don't seem to be getting well maybe it would be a good idea to open the drain and lower the water level.

Why do we grieve? We grieve because we have lost something we consider a vital part of our identity. Grief seems different than anger, jealousy, resentment or other negative emotions, but all negative emotions are different forms of fear, and all fear stems from one primary misconception: the failure to recognize the truth of our identity.

The experience of one's empowering true spiritual identity is the healing treatment that is life changing and permanent. The realization of our true Self brings about inner peace and joy within an unperturbed mind, and on the physical level, it releases our natural immune system to work unimpeded to keep us healthy.

CHAPTER 11

IMAGING OUR WAY TO HEALTH AND HEALING

The phrase, "fighting disease," has always seemed inappropriate to me. My mental image of a disease that needs to be overcome by fighting is a disease with imposing power and strength. Other ways of imaging the healing process might be more helpful. I have had my own personal experience of changing my mental imagery of an ailing joint, and seeing it respond.

What I Believe Is What I Experience

When I was in high school, I considered myself a pretty good football player and enjoyed everything about the sport. During the Spring training game of my junior year, I suffered an injury which badly damaged my right knee and ended my football career. I managed to mask my true feelings, but I was really quite angry and resentful, especially when I was not a part of the team which won the state championship my senior year! After several months, I recovered normal mobility of this knee, but the damage had been done and the joint was never stable.

Gradually over the years, it became worse with increasing pain and limitation. Finally during my mid-50s, I was unable to participate in any sports without marked discomfort and swelling; even walking was painful.

I consulted an orthopedic surgeon and underwent arthroscopic surgery. After several months, there had been no noticeable improvement and I was considering having knee replacement surgery.

I tried meditating, asking for Divine guidance about the meaning of this problem, and what to do about it. What I became conscious of was an unexpected and entirely different way of seeing this knee injury. For the first time, I realized its benefits. Without that injury I probably would have obtained a football scholarship to college, and majored in athletics. Instead, I took a different course and became an medical doctor, which has certainly resulted in an interesting life which is rewarding in many ways.

I had always thought of and referred to this knee as my "bad" knee. Now I had a different mental image. I began thinking about it as my "good" knee, and thanked it for the changes it had brought about in my life. The knee responded. The pain completely left and the swelling subsided. I can again play tennis and golf, and even climbed the mountain overlooking Machu Picchu, the famous Incan ruins in Peru.

The knee is not perfect, but is now about like the other one. Perhaps I can find a way to image perfection! I'm working on it. Maybe what is blocking my complete healing is my belief (mental image) in the inevitably of aging.

Gravity Versus Levity

Actually, words are simply symbols or images of our thoughts. I equate disease or illness with the word gravity, with all its implications of heaviness, seriousness, oppression, gloominess, and being weighed down. A life-threatening illness is often referred to as "grave," (and the outcome usually ends up in the grave.)

The antidote to gravity would be anti-gravity, or levity. This word brings forth images of freedom, lightening up, floating free, exhilaration, exuberance, effervescence, bubbling with joy. Norman Cousins found the connection between levity and healing. He was cured of his serious illness as he used humor and laughter to counteract the mental image of the weightiness of the problem, literally lightening up his attitude about his disease.[1]

Illness could be equated with being stuck in the mud of our own negative or fearful thoughts, and to heal we need to float free or elevate ourselves out of the quagmire binding us.

I am grateful for a scene from the movie, *Mary Poppins,* where actor Ed Wynn cannot stop laughing, and he becomes lighter and lighter until he floats upward to the ceiling. This high-spirited exuberance is contagious, and soon Mary Poppins, and her friend, Burt, and the children are all laughing and filled with glee, and they begin floating also.

This movie scene of getting lighter through laughter brings to mind the word "inspiring." Inspiration means filling the lungs with air, and this inspiration facilitates the delivery of life-giving oxygen to all the cells of the body. It also means being "in spirit." This latter definition reflects the healing idea of identifying with our enlightened, lighthearted, weightless spiritual selves rather than with our limited, serious, heavy-burdened, diseased, physical selves.

If we identify with our spiritual selves, there is a change in our attitude or vision, and the images we have created as blocks to healing do not appear so ominous. We float above them, so to speak, and are able to see the overall picture rather than being blinded by the stark, up close, images of illness. From this different vantage point, these images become less terrifying and we realize they are not insurmountable. We are able to see them as only scare-crows that we ourselves have created in our minds, and our fears have made them seem real.

To Heal, Use Love Instead Of Fear

There are distinct differences in the way patients undertake the fight for survival when faced with a life-challenging illness. It is really a difference in motivation, and depends on each patient's attitude, but the difference is all important. If the energy behind the effort to get well comes solely from an attitude of fear and its accompanying mental images of pain, physical deterioration, sacrifice, loneliness and dying, then the effort is exhausting and eventually self-defeating. This person thinks the problem is overwhelmingly serious and hopeless, and the immune system gets that message and begins to shut down, agreeing with the persons thought that defeat is inevitable. On the other hand, if the motivation behind the struggle to survive comes from an attitude of love of life and a desire to live fully, and all the glorious mental images associated with these thoughts, then one taps into an inexhaustible supply of life-giving energy which is invigorating, revitalizing, and healing. This sends a positive message to the immune system to get busy!

Jose's Story

One of my favorite patient-doctor experiences was with a man who changed his philosophy from that of fear to one of love for life. Jose was a man of Puerto Rican origin whom I saw at the VA Urology clinic in 1994. He had been found to have prostate cancer ten years earlier at the age of 64. At that time, he was living in New York City. Although the treatment choices presented to him seem rather inappropriate to me as a Urologist, I will relate them as he told me, which turned out to be accurate on checking his medical records.

Shortly following his diagnosis in 1984, he underwent an operation for the purpose of total removal of his prostate. However, at surgery the cancer was found to have spread to the lymph nodes, so the prostate was not removed. He was then treated with radiation. He did well for about two years, but then developed symptoms of urinary blockage. His prostate was again found to be enlarged and cancerous, and again the decision was made to attempt another operation to remove his prostate. This time the effort had to be terminated because of severe bleeding. The patient stayed in the hospital for three months, developed many complications, and almost expired several times. His doctors then advised intensive hormone therapy. He promptly developed pulmonary emboli (blood clots which lodged in his lungs,) and again he almost died.

Since the discovery of his cancer he had been fearful, but trusted that modern medicine could save him. Now he was exhausted, angry and disillusioned. He decided he had had enough, and requested that all treatment be stopped and that he be released. He went back to Puerto Rico because he wanted to enjoy being with his family and especially his grandchildren. He looked forward to working in his garden again. He wanted to spend whatever time he had left doing the things he loved and being in the company of those who loved him.

He did all these things, and when I saw him it had been eight years since he left the hospital; there had been no further treatment. He appeared completely healthy and was joyful and enthusiastic about life. On examination his prostate still felt like it contained cancer, and his blood test for prostate cancer (PSA) was still elevated. He was not interested in any treatment, however, and I was not anxious to prescribe any. Six months later on a return visit to my office, he was still healthy and the physical and laboratory findings were unchanged.

How does one account for the survival, and improvement in health of this man, in spite of the absence of medical treatment? My interpretation is that he gave up fear as his motivation for getting well. Jose was willing to accept whatever the future had in store, and he substituted as his goals the desire for joy and life. This positive choice must have encouraged his immune system to work more effectively to control the cancer. This message of determination and hope was validated and reinforced as he experienced the joy of being with his family, and the healthy, peaceful activity of gardening. Although he still has cancer within his body, he is controlling it, and it is not controlling his life. I would consider this a "miracle" of healing.

Taking Time To
Gather Our Forces For Healing

Recently the treatment of early prostate cancer has made a drastic shift. The PSA screening test and the availability of easily performed prostate biopsy using ultrasound guidance has dramatically increased the number of patients who are diagnosed with prostate cancer early in the course of the disease. These patients have a better chance of cure at this stage, and the treatment recommended by Urologists is usually radical surgical removal of the prostate or radiation therapy in an attempt to completely irradicate the prostate cancer. This plan certainly makes logical sense to me, and I adopted this strategy in my practice.

A patient who had the clinical findings on rectal examination of a distinct cancerous feeling prostate nodule would undergo a prostate ultrasound and needle biopsy of the prostate. If the diagnosis of this biopsy was found to be malignant, and there was no evidence of spread to distant locations within the body, then we proceeded to radical surgery or radiation. The PSA blood test on these patients was usually mildly elevated.

On occasion, especially when I was working at the VA clinic, the biopsy would be delayed for two or three months. Often I was surprised when I reexamined these patients, before biopsy or any treatment. Some no longer had the suspicious lump in their prostate, and their PSA levels had returned to normal. There was no doubt that something had definitely changed between my first examination and the second. The prostate biopsy was no longer indicated.

What could have happened to change the course of what had seemed to be an obvious early prostate cancer?

At the time of my initial examination, after finding an abnormal feeling prostate, I would discuss the possibility of cancer with these patients. I tried to present this unpleasant subject as positively as possible, talking about the high cure rate and implanting the idea that the body's immune system dealt successfully with cancer cells all the time. I tried to encourage the patient and convey to him that it was his own body that did the healing, but that our treatments could help if needed.

Now I am wondering if some of these patients did indeed have clinically detectable cancer but managed to heal themselves. There are quite a number of documented cases where, even after the biopsy shows cancer, no cancer was found in the surgical specimen when the prostate was totally removed a few weeks later.

From a holistic view, major invasive treatment that starts immediately after the shock of the diagnosis of a life challenging illness, with no time for mental and emotional adjustment, would appear to me to be ill-advised, subjecting the body to additional shock just when the patient (and his or her immune system) may be already paralyzed with fear.

It would be interesting to delay the major treatment of prostate cancer for a short period (4-6 weeks) after making the diagnosis, and then re-examining. Perhaps the treatment of other types of malignancies, such as breast or cervical cancer where observation and repeat biopsy is readily available, could be similarly delayed. I do not believe that this short delay would jeopardize the potential curative results of treatment, and during this time a vigorous supportive treatment program could be instituted to enhance the immune system.

During this interim period, I would recommend intensive therapy aimed at maximizing physical health, such as nutrition counseling, anti-oxidant vitamin therapy, exercise, life style changes, avoiding exposure to known carcinogenic substances, along with optimizing treatment of any other medical problems.

In addition, intensive mental health facilitation and counseling, such as that being done at the Getting Well center, would be an integral part of this pre-operative interval. This would have the specific goals of: (1) helping the patient overcome fear; (2) discovering motivations for living which may have been hidden by stressful life situations or relationships; (3) teaching positive imagery and relaxation techniques; and (4) encouraging him to become an active participant in the planning and implementation of treatment.

Many patients would not choose this delay, but for those who do, I can see only benefits from being better prepared for the proposed treatments, be it surgery, radiation, or chemotherapy. This treatment strategy need not only apply to cancer, but also to other illnesses where severely invasive therapy is being considered. Hopefully, there may be the occasional patient who manages to recover from cancer or other serious illness without the need for the proposed major invasive intervention.

I am suggesting that in the "fight against disease" we have concentrated our efforts on finding and using external sources of treatment, and we may have been overlooking the major force that can influence the outcome in a positive manner, and that is the healing intention of the patient. Without this, all other treatment efforts will have only limited success. It is time to re-focus our efforts. A patient can only become healed who (1) thinks he can, and (2) desires to get well; otherwise he blocks the most well-intended efforts of the physician.

CHAPTER 12

SEEING DISEASE
AS A MESSAGE

One might look at physical illness as a signal that something in the holistic (or whole) human being is "off the track." To state that in another way, something in the totality of the person is not functioning harmoniously, and this is showing up as a physical illness.

Nervous Breakdown/ Physical Breakdown

When a person has a "nervous breakdown" it is because the nervous system has become overloaded due to excessive worry, nervous stimulation or agitating life circumstances. The person's brain loses the ability to function as before. In common terms the nervous system "blows a fuse," bringing reasonable analytical thinking to a halt. The person is literally forced to take a break from whatever stresses have exceeded his mind-brain capacity, and to retreat into a period of rest and repair.

This person may choose to simply rest, and recover enough to return to his or her life activities unchanged, to again confront the same stresses in the same dysfunctional way, leading to another breakdown in the future. A more constructive way to spend the time following a period of rest and stabilization would be to seek to discover the self-defeating attitudes that could have been the precipitating factors. With medication and mental health counselors to assist, the patient may be able to unravel the puzzle of life that brought on the nervous breakdown, and avoid becoming trapped in the same dysfunctional behavior patterns.

In a similar manner, a person might consider physical illness as a "breakdown," sending a message that something is out of harmony. We are not simply bodies, but are the complete package of body, mind, emotions, and spirit, and the message may be coming from any of these areas. The illness is giving a signal, telling one: "Stop! Think about what you are doing! What are you thinking? What are you considering so important in your life that you are willing to sacrifice your health?"

Check The Foundation

Someone interested in renovating an old house would not be very smart to spend all the time, money, and effort required for this project without first having a good look at the foundation and making the necessary repairs. As with the house, a thorough examination aimed at uncovering the cause of our illnesses needs to begin with a careful look at our foundation structures, our underlying beliefs about ourselves.

Thanks to the advances of modern scientific medicine, most physical symptoms can be treated and controlled, at least temporarily. But instead of immediately assuming a physical cause and limiting our quest purely to the search for a physical cure, perhaps one should do a little "soul searching" of the other parts of his life that may be out of balance. Use what is available to treat the physical problem to remove the immediate danger, but don't stop there! Try to see the physical illness as a message to you, triggering one of the "land mines" underlying your mask of perfection, and providing an opening for you to explore. Your outer mask of health has been damaged, and something inside you has been exposed which thinks you are unhealthy or do not deserve health. Don't believe it! But don't ignore it either. Seek to find its false underpinnings and prove it wrong.

Henry's Story

I remember another VA patient who demonstrated an illness that could possibly have been thwarted years ago if the emotional history had been pursued and vigorous psychotherapy instituted.

Henry was brought to see me in the urology clinic to evaluate mild prostate symptoms. No significant urologic problem was found. The unusual finding was Henry's physical posture. His body was literally frozen in a completely straight position. He rode in a wheelchair in the reclining position with his feet straight out. He could stand with assistance, but could not bend. His arms were held rigidly at his side, his head erect and chin in. His diagnosis was rheumatoid arthritis, and he had been treated for years without any significant relief.

After my urologic exam was over, I asked the patient about his unusual condition. His answers were not very informative, but it struck me his position looked like someone standing rigidly at attention. I asked him about his military experience, and that is where his story became interesting.

Henry was of African-American ancestry and had been inducted into the military at the draft age of 18. He had grown up in a peaceful, rural environment, had an easy-going nature, and had never needed strong disciplinary measures. He was overwhelmed by boot camp. He had trouble taking seriously the shouted orders of the drill Sergeant, and was constantly being punished. Finally, he was forced to stand at attention for an entire day. The Sergeant would come by frequently, shout and curse at him, and physically strike him if he moved a single muscle. This punitive, demeaning treatment completely broke his spirit, and it wasn't long after this that his arthritic symptoms began.

All I could think of was that some military authority figure should tell him, "At ease, soldier!" Since I was the only one around, I did say that. I also reminded him that his old drill sergeant was now probably dead and buried. He looked at me with surprise and gradually I could glimpse a new understanding taking shape. He began to soften and to laugh, as if recognizing the connection between his rigidity and the humiliation of his youthful military experience. I hope he has been able to release himself from the emotional and mental chains which were binding him.

This patient undoubtedly has crippling rheumatoid arthritis, and had the laboratory tests to substantiate this diagnosis. However, I cannot help but believe the abuse he suffered and the resulting mental images he produced were causative factors in his illness. Perhaps modern psychotherapy could help uncover the buried fear and anger suppressed into his subconscious mind. Maybe then the treatment of his arthritis could be more effective.

First, Do No Harm

Most physicians of my acquaintance do not consider the Behavioral Medicine approach at the onset of a problem. This is unfortunate because a life-style change or mental correction at this point will certainly do no harm, and may result in preventing a lifetime of illness. This could save the person not only from future suffering, but from the expense and potential harmful side effects of drug therapy and the need for surgery, and allow him to be a positive contributor to society and the nations economy rather than a drain on the system.

Hypertension

One could choose any of a number of illnesses to demonstrate the connection between our thoughts and emotions and the manifestation of physical disease, but hypertension is an example of a diagnosis whose very name screams out that it is an illness related to stress. The treatment continues to be aimed at physically correcting the problem by diet, salt restriction, exercise, and medication. The common course for this disease of elevated blood pressure is a gradual progression toward problems of heart failure, kidney failure, stroke, circulatory problems, visual disturbances, and eventual death.

There has been a huge effort by the pharmaceutical industry to manufacture effective drugs, and this has been highly successful. However, these medicines are quite costly, (and profitable for the manufacturer), and there are many disabling and even fatal side effects. I have been to conferences where hours were spent discussing the most effective combination of these drugs and how to treat the side effects. No mention was made of the potential benefits of stress management or lifestyle changes.

Stress, or "tension," comes from struggling to obtain something one thinks is necessary for his or her happiness. In our society, this something is usually defined as some type of worldly success. Is it worth the price?

The population with the highest incidence of hypertension in this country are black males. I can imagine the frustration they feel and the struggle that is necessary for them to attain goals in life that are more readily available to others. Surely there must be a tremendous amount of buried resentment, hostility, and anger. Defusing this may be difficult, but finding inner peace of mind is not impossible either.

Another group of people who are commonly affected by hypertension and related cardio-vascular disease are those who are "experts" at control. They are usually quite successful in their chosen professions, but the tension and effort involved extracts a heavy toll.

If these 'controllers' can learn to relax this choking grip on life, and decrease the outpouring of adrenaline and similar stress related chemicals, then the tension in the small arteries also relaxes, and the force of the hearts contractions diminishes. The blood pressure becomes easier to control and frequently returns to normal.

There are many "mind-body" treatment techniques such as bio-feedback, training in mindful meditation, and psychotherapy that could help a significant number of these patients, and behavioral medicine is gradually becoming accepted as part of the treatment of this disease.

CHAPTER **13**

THE PLACE OF
PSYCHOTHERAPY
IN MEDICAL PRACTICE

In many ways, people are taking a more vital interest in what they can do for themselves to stay healthy. Just look at the numbers of joggers, the huge exercise industry, diet plans of all descriptions, health food stores, and numerous herbal health remedies. This is all well and good, and many people feel they are practicing a "holistic" method of healing because they are no longer depending entirely on their physicians to keep them well. But this is not "holistic" according to my understanding of this word, because, still, only physical solutions are being used, trying to correct the problems at the physical level and ignoring the deeper causative issues.

Psychotherapy literally means treatment of the mind. It is in the mind that shifts can occur and have a remarkable effect on the health of the individual. It is in this area that healing attitudes can replace previously held harmful, disease-producing attitudes.

Another Dimension Of Treatment

Changing one's mental imagery and modification of one's emotional response to the stresses of life does have an effect on the body's physiology. Getting Well, an out-patient facility in Orlando, Florida, believes this, and has many successful cases to prove it. It does not, however, make physical improvement its major goal. While cooperating with and encouraging physically directed treatments, it provides a unique environment for participants to tap the potent resources of their minds for getting well in the deepest sense.

It's founder and director, Deirdre Brigham, M.S., M.P.H., M.A., is the author of *Imagery for Getting Well: Clinical Applications of Behavioral Medicine*. This book is a comprehensive, authoritative and very readable treatise on the subject of behavioral medicine/psychoneuroimmunology (PNI).[1]

Since I have been associated with Getting Well, Inc. I have developed a long list of acquaintances who are living healthy and productive lives in spite of scientific medical prognoses that would have had them either dead or severely disabled long ago.

Some people are beginning to recognize their own dysfunctional patterns before they become physically ill, and are seeking psychological counseling before it becomes necessary to seek medical care. I think this is truly a great step forward.

At present, many patients must pay for this care themselves, and an increasing number find that option preferable to the alternative of long term, invasive medical care. Perhaps a time is coming when early psychological intervention will be recognized for its true value by third party payers.

Taking Personal Responsibility

I have indicated throughout this book that healing is primarily an inside job. This concept is a bit frightening, because most of us have become comfortable looking for cures that comes in pill form or through the ministrations of a healer of some sort, and we have little idea of where to begin our inside quest for health and healing. It is also likely to bring up resentment and even guilt in a person who is experiencing a severe illness, perhaps implanting an idea that this person has failed, and is somehow responsible for his or her illness. But let's try to look at this differently and on a brighter side.

Once a person has become convinced that the idea of personal responsibility may contain some truth, and has found the courage to accept a more active role in personal healthcare, then the doorway is opened for correction and healing. Now, he or she no longer has to see him or herself as a helpless victim, but can personally do something about it!

The most urgent need is a change of mind, a change in what we believe and the thoughts we think. Fortunately, this is where our greatest potential for change exists, and herein lies unlimited power. We may feel helpless when facing an illness on the physical or emotional level, but our mind is our own personal playground and laboratory, and we can change it anyway we wish.

Professional psychotherapists can be extremely helpful, but they are powerless to change anyone else's mind. They can guide us, and teach us valuable techniques, but in truth, we are our own psychotherapist!

For permanent healing to occur at any level, it must start in the mind. Healing occurs from the inside out, not from outside in. Just as a dentist does not put a cap on a tooth before first getting rid of the rotting portion of the tooth underneath, so we must clean out the decay in our minds. Just covering over the problem doesn't work!

The way sickness shows up on the physical level differs with each of us. Perhaps it has broken through at the "weakest link" in our outer protective cloak of innocence described in Chapter nine. This would be the area in our physiology that has been most eroded by the continuous eating away of harmful self-demeaning opinions and thoughts.

Fred's Story

I first saw Fred when he was about 75 years old. He was a tall, thin, Afro-American with very light brown skin, who complained of severe pain in his perineal area, (the crotch, or area between the anus and the genitalia), and difficulty urinating. Recent examination and biopsy had revealed prostate cancer. When I inquired about how long he had been hurting in this area, he surprisingly related to me the following story of long standing anger and frustration.

Fred had served as an enlisted man in the Army Air Force during World War II. He was stationed at a base in Florida for training. At that time the barracks were segregated, and the races were housed on different parts of the base. On Saturdays they had liberty, and rode into the nearby city on buses, which were also segregated. The buses stopped first at the "white" pickup area, and would fill up, leaving only a few seats in the back when they arrived at the "black" area bus stop and they were suppose to enter only through the rear door. The black soldiers were frustrated and angry at this system, but usually docilely accepted their plight.

One evening a few of these black soldiers refused to take this demeaning treatment any longer. They refused to enter the back door of the bus but insisted on boarding through the front door. The driver blocked their way and a violent argument arose, resulting in a fight.

The fight rapidly spread and developed into a full fledged race riot, including breaking into the armory, calling out the Military Police, and finally, forcibly subduing of the outnumbered black soldiers. During this melee, Fred had backed away and not entered into the fighting. He "hid" behind his almost white skin, hoping he wouldn't be noticed. However, he was cornered by some angry white soldiers who he remembers exclaiming, "Get him! He is one of them!"

Fred remembers being beaten severely, and while on the ground being brutally kicked in his crotch. He lost consciousness and woke up in the infirmary, swollen, bruised, and bleeding from his penis.

He developed a urethral stricture because of the injury, and required numerous painful urethral dilation procedures. He was later discharged from the army, declared unfit for duty, and was denied any disability payments. He was furious because he felt his injury was caused by the Army and they should accept the responsibility for it.

Fred devoted much of the rest of his life attempting to verify his claim for disability payments, through military, political, and civilian legal channels. He found that all records of this military "incident" had been carefully destroyed, along with any records of his initial injury and treatment! He has been "stone-walled" at every turn by total bureaucratic denial.

Over the years, Fred continued to have severe pain in the crotch area, and required many treatments including painful, invasive Urologic procedures because of infection and blockage and bleeding. The pain was a constant reminder to him of his unjust treatment and the futility of his efforts to receive compensation.

He said he wasn't surprised at all that he had developed prostate cancer, because that is exactly where he had been kicked, at what was, in his mind, the onset of his illness many years ago.

There is a tendency to jump to the conclusion that finding a just solution to this injury issue would solve all Fred's problems. However, I suspect that Fred's grievance probably goes deeper, and actually is a racial issue. He had always been dissatisfied about the very light color of his skin, and the feeling he was neither white nor black. He said his mother was a servant in a white home and was taken advantage of sexually by her white employer, who was his father. Fred was sorely frustrated about never being completely accepted by either racial community, and blames society for this perceived injustice. Again, it would be easy to stop here and blame an unjust social system for Fred's problems.

However, I get the idea that on an even deeper level, Fred has never really liked or accepted himself, using the racial issue as a scapegoat for his own emotional under-development. If he could develop the insight to look, Fred would probably find a rich vein of inner self-hatred and low self esteem which could be causative factors for a life of discontent.

The point is, even though in some cases such as Fred's there seem to be obvious connections between the physical manifestation of disease and the psycho-social history, usually no such direct connection is visible. Also, as can be seen from Fred's case, the deeper one probes the more one seems to move to a core problem which is quite different from the obvious surface issue. Invariably, if one goes deep enough, it is found that the problem is not something 'out there,' but is an internal error of perception.

A Tangled Web

We all have hidden grievances from the past, and we have many unhealthy thoughts daily based on these unhealed issues. The constant pounding of these negative thoughts finally affects our physical health. Tracing all these thoughts back to their source is not easy. Sir Walter Scott observed:

> *"Oh, what a tangled web we weave,*
> *when first we practice to deceive!"*[2]

He could well have been describing the mental origin of illness.

So when did we "first practice to deceive?" What was this first decision not to be truthful? I think the first lie that we told ourselves and accepted as truth was that we were independent beings, separate from each other and from our Source. This is our "original sin," or I prefer, the first error of humanity.

From this initial lie, each of us has woven our own web of self-deception, with one misperception building on another. Somehow we must find our way through this maze to the Truth about ourselves. Because of the "tangled web" of our self decep-tion, one cannot usually follow a single thread back and locate a single cause for an illness. After all, what we are manifesting today in our lives is a hodgepodge of all our beliefs, triumphs and tragedies, errors and omissions, victories and defeats, joys and fears.

One could rightfully observe that uncovering all our hang-ups and blockages, and then re-imaging them, seems like a long, arduous, process. It is not easy to revisit the scene of all our "sins" for which we carry shame and guilt, anger, or grief. It also seems that as soon as we have exonerated one deeply rooted problem another boils to the surface. It wasn't easy making all the mistakes in our lives, and the graveyard of our buried misperceptions is quite large. However, I have observed in my own inner explorations and that of others, there is a joyful sense of freedom as each new insight is discovered. This wonderful feeling of release encourages one to move on to the next step, and each time with a little lighter burden to carry.

A good example of this dynamic occurred recently to a friend who is cancer survivor. She has courageously dealt with many physical and emotional problems over the past five or six years since she received the diagnosis of breast cancer with bone metastases. Now 74, one of her long-held emotional triggers was the recurring memory of an abusive ex-husband who she felt had robbed her of much of the joy of life. She related how she was never willing to forgive him because she felt it would be like "letting him off the hook" for all the ways in which he had wronged her and her children. Suddenly one day, during a bout of angry resentment, it dawned on her that the unforgiveness was having no particular effect on him, but she was the one it was keeping on the hook of her volatile emotions. At that point, she was glad to let him and the anger go, and has not given her power away to these thoughts again.

CHAPTER 14

THE GRACE OF FORGIVENESS

As one continues the process of self exploration and correction, one invariably moves beyond the tendency of blaming others, and outside situations and things, and begins to see how one's own choices have been responsible for what followed. It is a recognition that, "Yes, these persons and things were a part of my drama and may have played the parts of my antagonists, but I am the one who is the creator and director of my own drama."

This is a major step forward, but it may leave one in the uncomfortable position of feeling guilty for making such a mess of one's life. Now comes the last, and perhaps the biggest step, and that is forgiving oneself.

Most of our errors in judgment we can't honestly justify. We simply have to admit that we made mistakes. Justifying these would simply be rationalization. It helps me to realize that, though some of my actions have been wrong, at the time, I was doing the best that I could with the tools I had. However, there is a more graceful way to self-forgiveness, and that is simply a process of remembering the truth of who and what we are.

True Forgiveness

I see True Forgiveness then as simply a correction of the basically flawed guilty image of ourselves. By forgiveness we change our belief about ourselves and are able to accept our God-created Magnificence.

One might say this is the height of pompousness, but in truth it takes great humility to admit that we have been unable to change what God created. To think otherwise is truly egotistical as it assumes we are more powerful than God.

I find great emotional relief in the idea that in spite of my apparent shortcomings and sometimes "sinful" behavior, I have not been able to change at all the Essence of my being. My willful behavior has not been powerful enough to overcome the Will of God, and therefore, although it has at times created a personal living Hell, thankfully, it has had no Real effect!

Remember the discussion about masks (false images we have made of ourselves and others): only what was hidden by them was the True Self. The outer cloak of innocence which we like to show off, and the inner shadow of self-hatred that we work so hard to conceal, are both false-faces. Forgiveness is the Graceful ability to see through these masks and not give them validity, *because they are not true!*

True forgiveness recognizes that all the sins of commission and omission which we feel we have been guilty of, or were inflicted upon us, have happened during a state of mind where we were mistaken about our identity. (You might say we are innocent because of temporary insanity!) All these things that we have done to another being were but directed at his or her masks, because we were oblivious to his/her true identity. No matter how horrible the crimes have been that the masked combatants perpetrated on each other, they had no effect on the True Self of either, which is eternally safe, perfect, unchangeable and beyond attack. Nothing has been changed or harmed in any way. Forgiveness seen in this way is like waking up from a terrible nightmare and realizing one is still safe, loving, and lovable.

Forgiveness of others is not a holier-than-thou gesture that we offer someone else thorough our generosity. Forgiveness of oneself is not an excuse for one's own errors. That would be like saying, "It was not really my fault" or "The devil made me do it." Forgiveness overlooks the superficiality of 'right or wrong.' It is a realization that the Creator made me and everyone else perfect, in His likeness; and even though in our confused state of mind we tried to destroy that perfection, our thoughts and actions that defied God's Will have had no real effect.

What a relief! There is no need for resentment, anger, remorse, guilt or self-flagellation. We can simply move on, this time trying to remember our own and everyone else's True Identity, and in this way avoiding future errors.

There seems to be a lot more hugging now, which wasn't part of our culture a very short while ago. Sometimes it is hard to hug someone who has "done us wrong," or someone with AIDS, or someone who is a convicted criminal, or who looks or smells or acts differently than what we are accustomed to. Perhaps a deeper recognition of the underlying spiritual Goodness in each other, and the willingness to put our superficial differences aside, is what this hugging is all about.

If you have ever watched a line of ants following some unseen trail across the sidewalk, you have probably noticed that they pause and touch, each time one meets another. It is as though they are saying to each other, "Oh, yes, I recognize you and you recognize me. We see the Truth of each other."

If we could do that, what a difference it would make in our society and our world. That is how we could start every day and every inter-action; the first thing we remember about ourselves when we wake in the morning, and the first thing we call to mind when we meet someone. "Hello, brother. Hello sister. I know who you really are."

Truth Or Consequences

When I was young there was a program on television called "Truth or Consequences." It was a rather simplistic game show where the host asked a question, and if the participant did not answer correctly he had to suffer some consequence, like a cream pie in the face. Perhaps life could also be called a game of Truth or Consequences, but the consequences here are much more severe, and they usually do not seem very funny.

In real life, Truth or Consequences is not really a game, but we play it every minute of every day. There is only one question: "Who am I?" Answering this question incorrectly, i. e., identifying as our limiting and fragile body and our imperfect egoic self, results in the consequence of experiencing a life of trials and tribulations, of disease and despair and death. The correct answer, identifying with our True Self, results in a joyful life of health and healing and inner peace.

When we are fully able to accept this Graceful gift of Forgiveness that comes with recognizing our True Identity, then we can gratefully experience the full meaning of the song, "Amazing Grace:"

> *"I once was lost, but now I'm found,*
> *Was blind, but now I see."*

CHAPTER **15**

CONCLUSION

Hope For A Better Tomorrow

The traditional health care system is too technical, too expensive, and has lost much of its ability to satisfy people's needs on a compassionate level. This system has discounted the intelligence of the patient, and unnecessarily shouldered the entire burden of healing and health. I believe patients, doctors, and caregivers of all description are ready for a change. Hopefully, in its place is evolving a system in which the patient assumes the role of informed decision maker, with the medical community offering expert assistance as teachers, counselors, technicians, and comforters.

We are seeing increased mutual respect and cooperation among the healing professions. There is a refreshing openness to new ideas, and an acceptance of the validity of a broader range of healing modalities. The arena of health care is expanding, considering the patient's well-being not only from a physical perspective, but recognizing and treating problems and deficiencies in the psychological, emotional, and spiritual realms as well.

This broadening of the concepts of health, healing, and disease goes beyond the individual person. The existence of states of dis-ease is identified in relationships, in society with its racial, ethnic, religious, nationalistic and ideologic conflicts, and in the sick environment. To be truly effective, healing must extend into all these areas.

Medical research can be more adequately funded using public funds, similar to our space exploration program of recent years. In that way, being less influenced by the profit motive with its need for immediate gratification, it can be free to search for a cause of illness and the potential for healing not only within the physical dimension, but anywhere that our consciousness is able to take us.

There is a tremendous future of hope for mankind as we move into the 21st Century. The 20th Century has been about fighting: fighting wars, battling social injustices, subduing nature, and conquering diseases. Let us hope the next century will be about healing our wounds and returning to wholeness. Instead of continuing our strategy of attack, we can embrace a new philosophy which will allow us to dismantle the cumbersome defense systems we have created, both outwardly in the world and mentally within our psyche. These defenses, erected because we saw ourselves as individual bodies in a fearful world of separation and isolation and specialness, have protected us at the cost of imprisoning and crippling us. Now it is time to throw off our shackles, to rise above this battlefield and see ourselves, each other, our planet, and our universe from a larger view reflecting our oneness.

We have for too long identified ourselves as severely limited. The next Millennium may be the time for making the giant leap to the universal recognition of our True Spiritual Identity, thus allowing the human race to exist on a higher plane where we can experience ourselves as one, free, and unlimited. At that level of heightened awareness we will accept miracles as the norm. There will no longer be the consequences of identity confusion that have plagued Mankind since we began this long, exhausting, physical journey away from Home. It has been a long winter. It's time for spring, and fortunately, like the seasonal springtime, we do not have to plan it or know how it happens. We sense its approach and look forward to this time of re-birth.

FOOTNOTES

Many of the references cited below have complete bibliographies identifying the original research information. I will cite specific articles only when it seems pertinent.

On occasion I may quote directly from a publication, but the context in which these quotes are used and the interpretations of the meanings are entirely my own.

CHAPTER ONE
1. Getting Well, Inc. *A behavioral medicine program for individuals with life-challenging conditions.*
    933 Bradshaw Terrace, Orlando, Florida 32806
    Phone: (407) 426-8662   Fax: (407) 426-8661
    Email: gtngwell@magicnet
    Website: www.magicnet.net/getting well

CHAPTER TWO
1. This is only a small part of the information contained in this eye-opening article about the prevalence of alternative medical practice in the United States: *New England Journal of Medicine;* David Eisenberg; Jan 18, 1993; 328(4); 246-52.

Page 29: These are numerous references listed in the extensive appendix of the comprehensive work, *The Future of the Body;* Michael Murphy; 1992; Jeremy P. Tarcher, Inc.; Los Angeles. Specific studies cited here included in the appendix of *The Future of the Body* are:

2. The positive effect of prayer on plants. *Psychic:* Miller, R.N.; 1972; 3:24-25.

3. A telekinetic effect on plant growth. *International Journal of Parapsychology;* Grad, B.; 1963; 5:117-33.

4. Some biologic effects of the "Laying on of hands." A review of experiments with animals and plants. *Journal of the American Society for Psychical Research*; 59:95-127.

5. Positive therapeutic effects of intercessory prayer in a coronary care unit population: *Southern Medical Journal*; Byrd, R.B.; 1998; 81:826-9.

6. A very thorough discussion can be found in chapter 10 of *Manifesto for a New Medicine*; James S. Gordon, M.D.; 1996.

7. *The Touch of Healing*; Alice Burmeister with Tom Monte; Bantam Books; Sept. 1997.

8. Lengthy discussion of this amazing historical event, and references: *A Holographic Universe*; Michael Talbot; 1991; Harper-Colins Publishers: NY, NY.

9. For thorough discussion and documentation of the placebo effect, see: *Harnessing the Power of the Placebo Effect and Renaming it "The Wellness Response."* Benson, H., Friedman, R.; 1996; Ann. Rev. Med. 47:193-99.

10. Additional references with extensive information and bibliographies on these fascinating subjects:

   The Future of the Body; Michael Murphy.

   Spontaneous Remission: An Annotated Bibliography of Selected Articles and Case Reports from the World Medical Literature; B. O'Regan & C. Hirshberg: 1990; Institute of Noetic Sciences.

   Spontaneous Healing; Andrew Weil, M.D.; 1995; Alfred A. Knopf, Inc.

CHAPTER FOUR
1. *A Course In Miracles*; Foundation for Inner Peace, Inc.: 1975.

2. *Journey without Distance*; Skutch, Robert; 1984; Berkeley, CA: Celestial Arts.

3. *Homeward to an Open Door;* Carol Howe; 1993. Carol's numerous *LifeWorks* audio and video tapes can be found at website: www.carolhowe.com.

4. Center for Attitudinal Healing: now located at
33 Buchanan Street
Sausalito, CA 94965

5. Network for Attitudinal Healing International, Inc.
P.O. Box 390129
Kailus-Kona, Hawaii 96739
Phone (888) 222-7205   Fax (808) 322-8894
Email: netattheal@aol.com
Website: www.attitudinalhealing.org

6. Monroe Institute
Route 1, Box 175
Faber, VA 22938-9749

CHAPTER 7
1. *A Course In Miracles* Workbook for Students; page 376.

CHAPTER 8
1. *A Course In Miracles* Manual for Teachers; page 75.

2. Institute for Noetic Sciences
475 Gate Five Road, Suite 300
Sausalito, CA 94965

CHAPTER 11
1. *Anatomy of an Illness;* Cousins, N.; 1979; New York: W.W. Norton.

CHAPTER 13
1. *Imagery for Getting Well;* Brigham, Deirdre D.; 1994; New York: W.W. Norton.

2. *The Lay of the Last Minstrel;* Sir Walter Scott.